STRENGTH TRAINING FOR WOMEN OVER 50

TAKE A FUN-FILLED JOURNEY TO TONE MUSCLES,
BOOST METABOLISM, AND IMPROVE BONE DENSITY
WITH EXPERT GUIDANCE

FRANCESCA RUSSO

CONTENTS

How Did We Get Here?   5

1. WHY DID STRENGTH TRAINING
   BECOME SO IMPORTANT TO ME?   11
   Meet me, Franny- Author and Narrator   12
   Hip Replacement Surgery?   14
   Developing a Plan!   15
   How I Met My Tribe Sisters.   17

2. IT'S TIME FOR A CHAT WITH MY
   TRIBE SISTERS   23
   What Did Your Doctor Say?   23
   The Hip Replacement Reveal   25
   Nora and Her Sore Muscles   30
   Robbie and Her Osteoarthritis   33
   The Speech   35

3. LET'S TALK MOTIVATION   39
   Why Do We Make Excuses?   42
   How to Stop Making Excuses   45
   How to Get in the Right Mindset   48

4. WE NEED A TRAINER!   51
   The Meet and Greet   52
   How Are We Going to Do This?   84
   Let's Go Shopping   89

5. I WILL PICK YOU UP AT 8!   95
   The Hell You Will!   95
   Am I Supposed to Pee and Fart?   97
   Don't Forget to Breathe!   103
   A Love-Hate Relationship With Your
   Trainer!   106

6. IS THIS HELL?   115
   My Eyelashes Hurt!   116
   It's Arm Day, and I Need to Lift My Wine
   Glass, Marco!   117
   Why Is My Ass Still Big, Marco?   118
   Damn! Franny Russo Just Bench Pressed
   60 Pounds!   120

7. DOCTOR VISIT DAY   127
   An Apple a Day?   128
   Hey Doc, It's Me, Franny   131
   Hello Doctor, Nora Here   134
   Robbie, the Doctor Will See You Now   137
   It Is Wine O'Clock Somewhere   140

8. IT IS TIME TO RE-EVALUATE   143
   Modified Exercises for Surgery Recovery   143
   Strengthening Exercises to Assist in
   Weight Loss   147
   What You Need to Know As You Age   154

9. CELEBRATE EVERY VICTORY   157
   It is Time to Plan the "Greece"
   Celebration   158
   Happy Birthday to Us and Hello Greece!   160

   Conclusion   167
   Resources   179

HOW DID WE GET HERE?

I would like to officially welcome you to the most unique strength training book for women you will ever read. Why? It is hilarious. It is relatable. It is motivational.

Additionally, it will actually improve your overall well-being. If you purchased this book, you may see similarities to my story. It is a common theme among us glorious older generations. I don't know about you, but I was always active in my youth. Then, you hit 50 and realize just how exhausted you are. Maybe you are a mother who has spent the last hundred years wiping noses and butts. Perhaps you are a spouse or partner who spent far too much time taking care of them and not you. All of these scenarios sound familiar because we all do it. We all give way more of ourselves to others than to us.

Regardless of your path, you may have had an epiphany like me. I just stopped moving in my life. No, this is not an exaggeration. I would do those easy things that required plenty of sitting and lifting my wine glass. I would get my groceries delivered; hell, I would get everything possible delivered. My prescriptions, take-out, clothing, nothing was off limits. Oh, and those nice leisurely walks I used to love taking after dinner no longer interested me. Why? Menopause happened, and stepping outside of air conditioning was not an option in my life.

I actually convinced myself that I had put in my time moving my body and deserved to spend my last years sedentary if I so chose. If I wanted to spend the next 30 or 40 years on my ass eating whatever I fancied, so be it. I worked hard my entire life, and this is my reward. Guess what? I was wrong.

My body enjoyed this lifestyle for a hot second, and then, after a year or two, things started seizing up, degenerating, and feeling unstable. I was winded, going up a flight of stairs. My knees would ache if I spent the day out shopping with my friends. I have a plan to live to be over 100, and the way my body was failing was proving to me I needed to change.

If you are similar to me, you have realized how much easier life will be with more energy, strength, and healthiness as we grow older.

The information I have read says that strength training is an amazing tool for transforming your body and maintaining your physical capabilities, which is good because I need that in my life. If you are a beginner, like me, seeking to build a sound foundation of strength, this book is your guide to unlocking your full potential.

In these pages, you'll discover the science behind strength training and learn how to incorporate basic exercises to get you started with great tips on staying motivated.

But this book is more than just a few examples of exercises aimed at older women who need to start safely and slowly. You'll also learn from an expert the importance of proper nutrition, rest, and recovery and how to incorporate these elements into the plan for your best results. With practical tips and advice from a top strength coach, this book will help you get the most out of your training and achieve the strength and fitness you need to feel confident and capable.

Let me introduce myself.

My name is Franny Russo, and I will celebrate my 55th birthday this year. I decided to write this book to help you, the reader, myself, and my lifetime friends Nora and Robbie, also known as my sister tribe. Besides, I love my life and want to live to be 101.

When I get off my couch, I am convinced I hear popcorn in the microwave. *Snap, crackle, pop!* Wait... that's a cereal commercial, but you get the idea. I am told this is because my ligaments are too tight. I find it hilarious to think that as I have aged, my muscles have become loose, and my ligaments have decided to tighten.

My boobs have sagged, and I now expect Herculean miracles from my bras. I now shop for "supportive" shoes and get excited about senior discounts. My hair has grayed, but I added a fun pink color to showcase my funny side. As I get older, the more I fart. We all do it. There is no escaping it; embrace it. My idea of a night out is to be back home in bed by 9:00 p.m., and I am okay with it. I love food, all the food. I can sniff sugar out seven miles away. I will plan an entire vacation around the food I can eat while I am there. I believe it is unfair that as I age, I am being asked to "watch my sugar intake." How about "No, thank you!"

More than anything, I am adapting to my new body, but it is failing me.

This book will be a journey with myself and my two tribe sisters, Nora and Roberta, as we realize the importance of having a strong body as we age. The trials, the tribulations, and the absolute blast we have is not something you will want to miss.

Remember, this book is packed with tools and knowledge you can use to improve your own quality of life. Discover all the benefits we unravel on our crazy, fun, realistic journey of strength training and life.

I have aimed to fill this book with valuable and practical strength training exercises that you, as a woman over 50, can not only gain from but want to use. It can be so disappointing to be excited about a new health voyage only to discover you are incapable of the exercises laid out for you. Trust me, if I can do these, so can you!

Join us for some concrete life skills, health solutions, strength training, and laughter. All this is wrapped up in the unique package of tribe sisters sharing the journey together. There is always room for one more.

1

WHY DID STRENGTH TRAINING BECOME SO IMPORTANT TO ME?

Hey there, it's me again, your trusted author and narrator, Franny! It is my time to dive in and tell you more about me. This chapter will be dedicated to all my details and why strength training is now a significant part of my life. If you happened to skip over the introduction, you might want to revisit that. Why? Well, it is kind of like meeting your friends at the movies, but you are the one who is always late. So then, you spend the next fifteen minutes asking what is happening so you can catch up. Trust me, it's worth the read!

MEET ME, FRANNY- AUTHOR AND NARRATOR

My name is Franny. I love red wine, dark chocolate, and salty men. Oh wait, that is my dating profile. Let me begin again.

I was born in Basilicata, Italy. Most have never heard of this village in the southern part of the boot because of how isolated it is. With almost no railway to speak of and no close airports, it has been closed off to the rest of the country. This isolation is a big reason it is one of the poorest parts, with only half of the residents employed (Bruno, 2022). My mother worked at a local market selling whatever we grew, and my father drank. He worked when it suited him. We left Italy when I was just a baby and settled in a small town in Kansas, U.S.A.

Our family would remain in this house for the rest of my childhood. It was your typical suburban home with wall-to-wall green shag carpet and paneled walls. Despite my mom being a clean freak, she, and all our relatives, were chain smokers (like most in this era), so the odor of smoke filled every corner of our home. Tupperware and CorningWare filled every cupboard, and the house sold with the same blue toilet we bought it with. My parents would never have any other children, and I witnessed their abusive marriage until I left home at 19. I would bury both of my parents and later sell this home.

I fall in love fast and easy, and my stack of marriage and divorce certificates is proof of this. Having been married four times and divorced four times, I have proven practice does not make perfect. I now admit that I am a free spirit and love living independently. It would have been less expensive to go to therapy in my 30s and discover this back then.

Throughout my many marriages, I would become a mom three times. To this day, they are my most significant achievement in life. I now live to embarrass them as often as possible. I believe it is my obligation as a mother. I have one amazing, career-driven daughter and two sons; one enlisted in the army, and the other a talented musician. None seem the least bit interested in making me a Gigi (my term for grandmother) anytime soon. I cherish the time we spend together, especially now that they are adults and on their own.

I worked a few menial jobs to make ends meet in my 20s and 30s, but I was exhausted from the financial stress. I wanted more for my family than I had. By more, I mean I wanted to be able to spend time and make memories with my children. My mom worked three jobs just to put food on our table, and I regret never having time with her. I thought I would have to sacrifice to better myself and my family. So, I went to school at 36 and became a licensed sex therapist. Okay, in all fairness, it didn't start out that way. I tried on a few hats first. First, I tried marriage counseling, and yes, I heard you giggle. I was great at it, yet I was still a bit of a cynic regarding gushy love stories. I am a great sex therapist because it is about making a person feel confident, free, and fabulous. I believe we all deserve that. I had never felt that my job was work, and it immediately improved my family's life.

I relocated to Arizona three years ago for the dry heat and to begin planning my retirement. I spend a crazy amount of time pressuring my tribe sisters to move here sooner rather than later and have finally convinced Nora to do so now.

However, as I reluctantly approach my 55th birthday, my doctor has told me I have osteoporosis and osteoarthritis in my hips and shoulders, but my hip is the worst.

HIP REPLACEMENT SURGERY?

I am headed for hip replacement surgery, and I am in denial. However, my doctor told me that I am sched-uled for this surgery in six months, and to recover quickly, I have work to do.

My doctor said that I must seriously reconsider my strength and conditioning routine. What routine? He would also like me to reevaluate my nutritional needs because if I can eliminate some weight before surgery, the recovery will be less painful.

What I heard: You are a fat lazy cow. You eat everything in sight. You are so unhealthy that you will be in pain forever once we do this surgery.

Retirement is knocking on my door, and I have no plan for this part of my journey. The plan I had always envisioned for myself and my tribe included living in Arizona, lounging by the pool, sipping umbrella drinks, and having glorious vacations. Instead, now I am staring at surgeries and walkers.

I feel a group chat is needed to discuss this doctor's visit, but I am aware I just need to bitch about the audacity of this man. A second opinion, please!

DEVELOPING A PLAN!

This is now the critical time that I need a plan. Without it, I will bail and crawl into that cozy nest of a cocoon I refer to as my bed. We all do it in times of difficulty. Screw it; I am not participating. I'll be in my blanket fort if you want to find me!

I also need reliable resources. Having a plan in front of you is one thing, but you might as well wipe your butt with it without a way to work it.

I realize that sounds harsh, but it is true. How often throughout your life have you read a mantra? For example, "Breathe, exhale, relax, and let go." Sounds amazing right? Well, I always read those and think, that sounds beautiful, but how? So explain to my busy brain exactly *how* to let go?!?

This situation is no different. Having that plan is a wonderful and vital first step, but you constantly feel so much more prepared if you know what resources to lean on as well. I am also going to need so much support.

I have never, ever in all my whole life, entered a gym, placed one finger on a weight, and I have been known to mock those who do. I firmly believe that every human should be allergic to spandex and that all workout gear smells like puddle water. While on a roll, can someone please explain the "need" to drink from a sports bottle when working out? Thousands to choose from, and some even decorate their names in glitter across the side. I just do not understand. Is this in case you misplace it, and someone can holler, "Is this Tiffany's sports bottle? Is Tiffany on the elliptical?"

I am aware I need to address what I shovel into my face. Do I want to? Hell no. But I must reach my goal of living to be 101 years old. Again, I am still figuring out how but I will begin with strength training first. Now, back to my blanket fort!

HOW I MET MY TRIBE SISTERS.

As mentioned, my family moved from Italy to the United States when I was just a baby. The home we moved into is where I stayed until I left to get married the first of many times. So I was the first of the tribe sisters to live on our cul-de-sac.

Meeting Nora

The day that Nora moved to our street, I was only two years old. I remember the story my mom told me about that day Nora moved next door. It was February, and Kansas was hit with a freak blizzard. Their moving truck was stuck, buried to the tires, and blanketed with over 13 inches of snow. So many neighbors were out shoveling and trying to help when my mom offered to bring Nora over to play with me so the family could tend to things. Unheard of today, but in the 1970s, parents thought nothing of allowing another woman to watch over their child. A beautiful young girl, braids tied with purple bows, clutching a stuffed dog. I still have a photo of us that my mom took that day, and our brightest smiles are plastered across our faces.

I do not remember a time in my life without Nora in it. We lost our first teeth together, studied for exams together, shopped, got our periods together, went to dances, and cried when boys broke our hearts and when we gave birth. She was a bridesmaid at every single one of my weddings. We buried our parents within a year of one another. We have been each other's lifelines through some very dark times.

Nora always looks on the bright side, and is full of sunshine. She appears to have it all from the outside. From the inside, that is not always the case, I know when Nora needs a hug, a vacation, or wine. I appreciate her and all she brings to my life. I should also mention that Nora is the workout ass-kicker of our group. I swear she was born in spandex, and I loathe her for it most days.

We live very different lives but respect what we bring to each other.

Meeting Roberta (who only answers to Robbie)

Roberta entered my life like a breath of fresh air, but I could tell she had an edge. I was 10 years old and remember it was in the dead of heat in August. The yellow house on our street went up for sale, and a red-sold sign streaked across it within two days. Places didn't go up for sale often in our small town, and when they did, people talked. Who was moving in? Nobody had a clue.

I was fast asleep on a Saturday morning, a rare cool breeze kissing my cheeks, blowing in through the open window. I was suddenly startled awake by a loud truck rumbling down our road, followed by many voices. As I rubbed the sleep from my eyes, I peered through the sheers, and that is when I saw her.

Flaming red hair and the most incredible rock band t-shirt (The Rolling Stones) the coolest I had ever seen. I jumped to my feet and ran into the kitchen, hollering at my mom that the new family had arrived. She, of course, was way ahead of me, announcing that she had already introduced herself. An American military family was moving into the home across the street from Germany. She told me to be kind to the young girl because her father had recently died. When I asked how he died, I was just told it was because he was in the military. I am sure this was the explanation given to me because of my age. I don't know if I understood the depth of this at that moment. I ate breakfast fast, called Nora, and we made plans to go meet the new girl.

We walked straight up to her, "Hi, I love your t-shirt," I said.

She kept her eyes focused on the ground while saying hello back. "My name is Roberta, but I only like being called Robbie." The young, shy girl replied.

Without giving it any thought, Nora gave her a hug. I followed suit. That group hug cemented our tribe for life. Three young girls, strangers in a sense, just knowing that one was hurting and needed some love, our group hugs would remain our signature for a lifetime.

My friendship with Robbie is respected because she always "tells me like it is." Most fear doing this as if I will freak out, scream, yell, and never speak to them again. Past behavior is a bitch, isn't it? Robbie stands her ground with me, always has, and never backs down when I need to hear the hard shit.

For example, she knew two husbands ago that I needed to be free and single, but I refused to listen. She now has claimed to not only stand up in church if I dare to marry again—when they ask if anyone has any reason this couple should not marry—but states she will be naked and chanting. I believe her with my entire being.

Over our lives, we met plenty of girls, both young and old, but no one ever "fit." They always tried to pit us against each other when all we wanted was to grow our circle. I have been blessed and am beyond grateful for my tribe sisters. We have grown and gone through it all.

2

IT'S TIME FOR A CHAT WITH MY TRIBE SISTERS

Here we all are, approaching 55 and with different health concerns. The first step in our plan was to book an appointment with our doctors to discuss our individual needs. We have now met with them and have been given all the details we need to get started. We agreed to get together for the weekend, and I am anxious to hear about what is up with my girls and fill them in on my journey.

WHAT DID YOUR DOCTOR SAY?

Despite not being excited about the topic of conversation, I was ridiculously giddy to spend the weekend with my tribe sisters. I kept the social activities to a minimum because my damn hip was flaring up, and

Nora was in the process of packing for her big move down here to Arizona. Her stress hives are sure to wreak havoc.

Nora would be the first to arrive as she drove to bring more things for her new home. She and I would then head to the airport and pick up Robbie before dinner.

I actually found myself pacing and obsessively watching the clock. I always felt a piece of me was missing when I wasn't surrounded by my tribe. Finally, my very weak bladder forced me to make another bathroom trip, and it was then I heard tires against the gravel in my driveway. I wiped as if my life depended on it, and with my pants still undone, I bolted out the front door, swirling Nora around in circles.

"Jesus Franny, are your pants open?" She questioned as I burst out in laughter.

"Oh, who cares! Just give me a hug already," I clambered back, overly excited to see her.

As we headed into the house, she instantly noticed my limp and asked how bad the pain was. I was great at glossing over these things with everyone but Nora because the nurse in her always called out my bullshit. "Bad enough I sat my ass in a doctor's office and now here we are!"

We quickly dropped Nora's luggage off at the house and headed to the airport. We made signs stating—*Pamela Anderson, Your Sisters Are Here*—because we always made hilarious signs when picking each other up at airports. She spotted us, and the screams started. Crowds turned their heads, and you would have thought a high school cheer squad entered the building. Yes, we are like this every time we find our way back to each other.

Together again, whole once more, and ready to discuss the retirement chapter of our lives.

Back at my house and settled into our best pajamas, all our favorite food and snacks and wine flowing, we were ready to dive in.

THE HIP REPLACEMENT REVEAL

"My doctor is a piece of shit who hates fat women, so I think I need a second opinion!" I blurted out before everyone even got seated. Robbie spewed wine out her nose, and Nora "tsked tsked" me.

Nora insisted I start from the beginning, demanding test results and actual diagnosis.

"Fine." I groaned like a hormonal teenager.

Before all meeting up, our tribe agreed to 100% full disclosure and no holding back. We had to be completely honest with one another to make a plan that would work for all of us. We had to be truthful if we wanted to be accountable and healthy.

"I have been hiding my pain from you both for a long time." I blurted out before my courage dissolved into thin air. I was boldly honest and told them I was afraid to find out what the pain was from, convinced it may be bone cancer like my grandmother had.

I can tell them that pain impacts every part of my day now, and I have noticed that I will avoid certain activities based on how bad my pain is at that time. That I average five hours of sleep because pain wakes me constantly. My pain ultimately made me decide to retire early, and I still feel defeated.

"I am turning 55 and my body feels 85," I confess, feeling a lump in my throat and tears stinging my eyes.

Throughout the years, my tribe knows something is serious in my life if I cry. However, I do not like to feel vulnerable the way crying makes me, so if it happens, shit is getting real.

"Franny, I am so sorry you have been struggling and we didn't notice. We will do better," Robbie says as she wraps her arms around me. Nora is quick to chime in, wanting to know what the doctor has said, and I can see concern all over her face.

"Well, it seems I am lucky to have both osteoporosis and osteoarthritis in all of my joints, but it has spared my spine so far, and it seems my hips and shoulders are the worst. Hold onto your knickers, girls. It gets worse. My left hip has gone to shit, and it needs to be replaced. My surgery date has already been set. Six months from now, I will go under the knife and become a bionic woman.

The girls know I attempt to use humor to cover up when I am anxious as hell, and it is all over my body language at this moment. I cannot sit still and shake as I pour my second glass of wine.

Robbie asks a logical question about how I got osteoporosis. Great question, and one I did ask the doctor. "He told me there are many factors that influence this, from hormones to genetics, but for me personally, it is likely because both my mother and grandmother had it, and my body mass index has been over 19 for over 20 years (NHS, 2017). So yup, my guilty pleasures all these years did not help."

Robbie quickly followed up with another question about how common are hip replacements?

"Buckle up ladies, I am now practically an expert on this topic," I bragged as I pulled out my notes from the visit I had with my doctor.

I told them I was shocked when he said that almost 850,000 hip replacement surgeries were done yearly in the United States alone (Levine, 2022). What was even more shocking to me was just how far this surgery has come. My surgery would only take an hour; I would be home that same day if no complications were encountered. "I just about pooped my drawers right there, when he told me I would be sent home that day, ladies."

With all her medical terminology and advanced jargon, Nora quickly assured me that this was normal. Gone are the days of ripping the bones from your body, replacing them with titanium, and leaving you in bed to rest for weeks. Nope, now you are expected to jump from that bed within hours and begin training for the Olympics; I shit you not!

I wrap up my chat session with the ladies, telling them my doctor insists I meet with a strength and conditioning coach immediately. He claims my rehabilitation will be faster and less painful if I strengthen my muscles. Being diagnosed with osteoarthritis is for life, and strength training is a great way to alleviate the painful symptoms that come with it.

"I looked at him sideways ladies and told him straight up this was not going to happen because most days I can barely lift my coffee mug."

Nora wrapped her arms around my shoulders, knowing my mood was fear-based, and insisted the doctor was correct. "Franny, we all know how you feel about working out, but hear me out."

She went on to explain that it is, in fact, our muscles that support these aging joints, and the stronger our muscles are, the less stress we place on them. Nora wanted me to understand that she knows those with osteoarthritis fight pain daily. She also wanted me to know that being sedentary will cause everything to cease up and create more pain when you try to move. My logical brain understands this, but my pain tolerance does not.

I told Nora that my doctor explained that strength training could help tone down joint pain and muscle stiffness, help with bone strength, and support a healthier weight. He pointed out that it also has the ability to improve my gait speed and my stability, especially after my surgery (Comprehensive Spine Institute, 2021).

So there you have it, ladies, my diagnosis in a nutshell. If I am being honest, the surgery scares the shit out of me, but so does how quickly my pain escalates. I have so much more living to do and cannot do it with this much pain. Dieting, on the other hand, well, there must be another way, yeah?

At the same time, Robbie and I turned our gaze to Nora and motioned for her to spill it.

NORA AND HER SORE MUSCLES

"First, let me say how sorry I am, Franny, that you are facing this diagnosis and surgery," Nora begins, patting my knee. Nora takes a huge breath and a sip of wine, and the tears start.

We rush to her side, and, to be quite honest; we are shocked by this because Nora isn't one to fall apart unless it is serious. Robbie is first on the scene to reassure her. "What is it? You are scaring me," Robbie says, wrapping Nora in a tight hug.

"Girls, I am okay, I am not leaving this earth anytime soon, but I need to stop denying what a bloody mess I am," Nora tells us that the doctor told her she is in great physical shape for her age. None of this shocks us; she lives for exercise and eating right. Nora mentioned to her doctor how she is more stiff and sore in the morning, but all her blood work is fantastic. He suggested she visit a strengthening coach who can help her adapt to new routines as she ages.

"Honestly, it is my mental health that is in the gutter right now and it is affecting me physically," Nora continues, wiping tears from her cheeks. I rub her back gently, reminding her we are here to support whatever she needs.

"I just don't understand how you can do something your entire life and then wake up the next day, and the world tells you they no longer need your services." The tears flow faster now as she struggles to control her emotions. "I am not done being a mother. I am not done being a nurse." Nora sounds angry, frustrated, and so disheartened that society tells her it is time to hang up all her hats.

If there is one thing we can agree on in this room, it is that being told that it is time to buy a rocking chair and learn to knit by society will never fly with this tribe! I have to reassure my girls if I am going to cheer them up at all. "I'll drink to that," Robbie says, raising her glass as if making a toast.

Nora's doctor has set her up with a therapist here in Arizona to help her with this new transition. "He realizes the toll this is taking physically and mentally and wants me to talk to them about empty nest syndrome." I, being a therapist of the sexual kind, am still very much aware of this condition and encourage Nora to jump at this chance for help.

Robbie questions, "I don't understand, am I heartless that I am enjoying this time to myself?" I jump in to give a brief overview and allow both women to understand that empty nest syndrome is simply a massive ball of grief we experience as our children leave. If we deal with it as it comes, we tend to be okay, but if our worlds have been consumed with parenting—and only parenting—we can be left grieving our sense of self. It can take up to two years to heal from this type of grief (Department of Health Services Victoria, 2012).

"Okay Nora, we will get this sorted. How are you feeling about tweaking your strengthening workout routine?" Robbie asks.

Nora perks up a bit because if there is anything she is passionate about, it's health and exercise.

"I took a hot minute to feel sorry for myself because, at the end of the day, you are being told you need to slow down a tad, but I'm also in fantastic shape and I can't wait to do this with my girl's!" she answers while jumping up and down like a mouse on steroids.

"Listen ladies, if I am being completely transparent here, my mental health has scared me this past year and I don't want to stay in this dark place," Nora continues. "I have done lots of research, and I want to dive deeper into this new therapy. I also want to learn more about how being physically strong can help keep me be mentally strong, and I want this for all of us." She is now more serious but her calm self once again, looking each of us in the eye.

"I am not just blowing smoke up your asses ladies. The proof is in the pudding," Nora spouts.

I can tell she is about to get super passionate and excited because she has jumped to her feet again. My current trainer told me last week that it is proven that strength training helps our bodies control hormone dumps, which in turn helps control our emotions (MacPherson, 2023). In addition, he read to me a study that showed anxiety and panic attacks dropped by 20% in a group that used strength training as a way to cope with these issues (Gordon et al., 2020).

We could finally see the spark Nora typically displays across her beautiful face, so I took that chance to join in. "Nora, my wonderful friend, this sounds like what we all need!"

Both Nora and I slowly turned our heads to face Robbie. She knew it was her turn next.

ROBBIE AND HER OSTEOARTHRITIS

"Well, girls, what can I tell ya? It isn't nearly as bad as I expected," she said, blatantly avoiding eye contact. The only time she ever did this was when she had shit to say but wasn't prepared to face the fallout. "We all know I have been under a shit ton of stress since coming out to the kids, and I haven't been dealing with any of that the way I should do," Robbie explains, her voice shaking just a touch.

I try to interject here because I can always tell when Robbie is about to say "screw this" and bolt. So I started asking some easy lead-in questions to keep her invested and calm her down simultaneously. "Why not start slow and let us know what your bloodwork showed," I probe a little.

"No surprise there, I am officially prediabetic, and my doctor—wait for it—thinks my drinking is an issue." Robbie is getting angry, and I know this because she has a vein that swells straight down the middle of her forehead. "Oh, it gets better; the twat also told me I have osteoarthritis. There you have it ladies, my idiot doctor thinks I'm a huge whale, an alcoholic, and I'll be using a cane in no time!" She yells out, half in tears, as she storms out of the room.

Nora rushes off after her while I take a moment and honestly let everything soak in. What in the "actual dirty martini is going on here?" The tribe is a hot mess, and I need to rally the troops.

"Ladies, I will need you back in here asap!" I bark, prepared to pull out the big guns. But I cannot be pulled into the emotion as I watch Nora lead Robbie back into the room by the hand. I need to stay on track.

THE SPEECH

Having the tribe seated in front of me, I grab my notes. "I know you will both be shocked to know this, but I have prepared a bit of a speech with the help of my doctor."

I encourage you, the reader, to take note of this awe-inspiring, educational, and loving talk. You didn't think we would leave you out... no way!

As women, the physical and mental health issues we face at this time in our lives are common. However, the most significant problem is that we tend to ignore them. We are so busy caring for everyone else that we put ourselves on the back burner. This is the mentality we need to change immediately. In order to enjoy the journey of retirement, grandchildren, or travel, we need to take care of our health.

For example, if you are diagnosed with prediabetes, the lifelong damage of diabetes—primarily to your kidneys, blood vessels, and heart—could already have started. We need to remember that progression from prediabetes to type 2 diabetes isn't predestined, but you need to take it seriously (De Filippis, 2022). Yes, it means changing our diets to eat healthier foods and lowering our body weight, but ladies, I believe hitting our goal age is worth it!

Osteoporosis is up next and not a fun one to deal with. It can cause our bones to be frail and brittle—two things we are not! I am serious, ladies, so weak, in fact, that a coughing fit could cause a rib fracture (Mayo Clinic, 2021).

When I asked the doctor what osteoporosis was, he told me it occurs because creating new and healthy bone doesn't keep up with losing old bone (Mayo Clinic, 2021). So, I asked him, "How do we strengthen these weak bones?" Apparently, some medications can help restore and strengthen them. Great foods we will talk about later, but strength training is vital.

All right, ladies, what do we know about osteoarthritis? I discovered it is the most common type of arthritis, and most call it the "wear and tear" disease. It eats away at our joints and mainly affects our hips—as I know all too well—knees and hands. So again, I asked my doctor what causes this, and I was told the cartilage—the mushy bit between our joints—breaks down and can cause our bones to change shape (Centers for Disease Control and Prevention, 2020).

There you have it, ladies, our three most significant ailments. In addition, our mental health has taken one big jump into a mountain of laundry we do not want to touch. You know the kind of laundry I'm talking about, right? It has been accumulating for weeks, everyone in the house is down to their last pair of underwear, and it is 7:00 p.m. on a school/work night. In the best-case scenario, you can get two loads of basics done by midnight, but all you want to do is run to Walmart, buy new granny panties, and call it a day.

I am here, standing on my soapbox, demanding we deserve better. I, the one who hates gyms, hate working out and hates dieting. I, the one who puts herself last just like we all do. It is our time, ladies, every last one of us.

If you hear one message from this amazing, hilarious, yet serious book, it is this: Nobody but you will do the work necessary to live a long and healthy life. That time is now, so buckle up bitches. We are about to get our best selves on!

3

LET'S TALK MOTIVATION

Motivation is the driving force or inner desire that pushes us to take action, set goals, and pursue our aspirations. The internal or external stimuli excite us and sustain our behavior toward achieving a particular goal. There are numerous sources from which motivation can arise, like personal beliefs, needs, desires, social influences, rewards, and consequences. Motivation is a critical element that significantly affects the outcome of our endeavors, and it plays a crucial part in shaping our personal and professional development. "Sounds easy right? Wrong! Motivation is one of the toughest obstacles we all face when making a big life change,"

"Scaring me into strength training, I believe, was my doctor's goal all along, yet here I am already finding a hundred reasons why I don't need any of it," I confided to both of them.

"We love you so much, Franny, but knowing what you are facing with your hip replacement, being in excellent shape is crucial. I am sure your doctor told you that it will drastically improve your pain levels and speed up your recovery, right?" Nora states.

Robbie interjects, "Listen, I am not one to offer advice, but I am going to need you to sit down and listen. You and I both know I don't want to participate in gym activities any more than you do. Slapping that spandex on my ass doesn't make me feel warm and fuzzy. But yet, what I know for sure is that you need this. Hell, I need this.So, I say, let's all do it together," Robbie states.

I truly have the best friends a woman could ask for. Knowing that both of you are ready to jump on this strength training bandwagon fills my heart. You know me, I don't tend to be sappy, but I feel so grateful to have you, ladies. I must be honest with myself and admit that I wouldn't even attempt this if it weren't for you both. Having your support while I face this obstacle will not be forgotten.

Robbie chimes in, "Have you ever asked yourself why, though? Like why do we self-sabotage the things that will bring us health and comfort? I swear, it seems like there are times we don't believe we are worthy of it. Franny, I know you are frightened of the surgery, but despite us dreading strength training, I know we will come out of this better and stronger,"

I agree with you both about the motivation side of things. Hands down, this will be our biggest obstacle. I invested a lot of time thinking about who could assist us the most with this. I reached out to my therapist because I knew she had a contact who was a sports psychologist. I thought, who would better explain why our brains refuse to participate in physical activity?

Initially, I was nervous to meet with him. I could only imagine some doctor/therapist coming at me in workout gear and a clipboard. Does a sports psychologist make you exercise while they provide therapy? I was entirely ignorant of what lay ahead and was about to get into, so I am so glad I met with him. He was nothing short of amazing and did offer me some clarity in this area. My first question was, why do we do this? Why do we seek reasons to skip physical activity, such as strength training?

WHY DO WE MAKE EXCUSES?

He gave me an entire list of reasons you will find below:

- **Lack of motivation:** The most common reason people find excuses to avoid working out is a lack of motivation. They may not have a clear goal or purpose for working out, making it difficult to stay motivated and committed. Without a plan and goals, you will always talk yourself out of working out and go straight to the couch, wine in hand.
- **Fear of failure:** Some may fear failing at workouts or not seeing the desired results. This fear can lead to procrastination and avoidance of working out altogether. It could be as easy as recalling a bad experience at a gym, or maybe you were injured while working out. You will now need to put that in the past and work toward the future.
- **Busy schedule:** We all have busy schedules and may feel that we don't have enough time to work out. We might use this as an excuse to avoid working out, even if we could make time if we prioritized it. All it takes is looking over your current daily schedule and finding that

space. Maybe you typically spend 45 minutes scrolling social media to unwind. Perhaps you fall onto that couch after work and don't move for two hours. It is merely taking time from activities that aren't beneficial to you.

- **Physical limitations:** Some may have physical limitations that make working out difficult or uncomfortable. This may include chronic pain, injuries, or disabilities. We must know that strength training can help decrease your pain once you start.

- **Lack of confidence:** Some of us may lack confidence in our abilities to work out, leading us to avoid it altogether. They may feel intimidated by gym equipment or other people working out around them.

- **Perceived inconvenience:** We may view working out as inconvenient because of the time commitment, the need to travel to a gym or workout facility, or the perceived effort required. Again, this comes down to prioritizing your health and working out.

He followed up with this: "These are just partial reasons why you may find excuses to avoid working out. It is crucial to recognize the key reason behind your justifications and strive to overcome them to establish a regular workout regimen," the therapist told me in closing.

"I met with him three more times before discovering what my ultimate issue is. Okay, issues—plural. It turns out that for me, it is a lack of confidence and a fear of failure. Two things about my feisty personality are that I hate to feel less than or not good enough and entering foreign territory, like a gym, makes me feel beyond vulnerable," I reveal.

Then Robbie pipes up, "Wow, this really resonates with me on numerous levels. I too struggle with the confidence part but I definitely fit into the 'inconvenience' bit. I really value my time and giving up a set amount each day for strength training makes me anxious, wondering what I have to give up to make it all work."

"For me, I would say I fall into the busy schedule and fear of failure categories. I always overschedule myself and barely find time to eat. Making this a priority is what changed my mindset. I have taken care of everyone my entire life, so taking time for my health is not selfish. It is a necessity," Nora chimes in.

So, then the question is, how do we change this? How do we find that motivation and throw away all the excuses?

HOW TO STOP MAKING EXCUSES

"I had a long chat with the sports psychologist about this. He did reassure me that the majority of people find themselves making excuses to avoid strength training. He confirmed that this is a common struggle for many people. Below are a few tips that will help extinguish some of the excuses:

- **Set achievable goals:** This can be one of the most common reasons people make excuses to skip the gym is because they feel overwhelmed or intimidated by the idea of working out. To combat this, set achievable goals that you can work toward, such as working out for 20 minutes a day or completing a specific number of reps or sets.
- **Find a workout buddy:** Exercising with a partner can help you in staying committed to your fitness routine and motivated to go to the gym. Plus, it can be more fun to work out with a friend! I feel blessed that my friends are joining me on this journey.
- **Create a routine:** Make strength training a part of your daily routine, just like brushing your teeth or taking a shower. Develop a routine by

scheduling your workouts for the same time each day. This helps to form a habit.

- **Eliminate distractions:** Avoid checking your phone or getting caught up in other distractions while at the gym. This will help you stay focused on your workout and less likely to make excuses to leave early.

- **Reward yourself:** Create a system of incentives to motivate yourself to adhere to your strength training program. This could include anything from a massage to a new pair of fancy shoes. Having something to look forward to can help motivate you to stay on track," Franny says in closing.

"These are all fantastic ideas and I would be lying if I didn't state that I will be using all of them. Working out with friends, check. Setting reasonable goals, I will rely on our trainer for that. Starting a regular routine will be necessary for me in order to stick to it. Lastly, rewarding myself is one of my favorite things to do," Robbie admitted.

Nora snickered, "Do I need to remind you both have laid some pretty ridiculous excuses for me in the past? My alarm didn't go off. My car won't start. I can't find my keys, shoes, purse, phone... I have two favorite excuse stories you both gave me."

"Franny, do you remember that time you agreed to be my plus one for a co-worker's wedding? I reminded you all week and then that morning you tried to tell me you couldn't come because you contracted an allergy to flowers. Not one specific flower, but all flowers, or so it seemed, and it magically appeared over the past few days just before the wedding," Nora says, rolling her eyes.

"Oh, I remember. I did tell you weddings make me nauseous now, but you wouldn't hear it. I learned my lesson not to use any medical excuse because you will call my bluff," I laughed.

Nora continued, "Robbie, I wonder if you recall that time you offered to pick me up from the airport? I was coming home from visiting family and you made it clear that picking me up would be no problem. After three very long hours, you finally texted me back. Across my screen, I saw, 'Sorry, turtle sick at vet emergency room, and I couldn't have rolled my eyes any harder. I am just as much an animal lover as the next guy, yet I knew you didn't even own a turtle."

"I never specified that it was *my* turtle, just *a* turtle. I happened to be babysitting it for a friend and you cannot let someone's pet die on your watch," Robbie said in her own defense.

"All I am saying is that I want to get to the bottom of our excuses, so I am not ready to ship you both off to a deserted island. We need to all be on the same page because I don't want to be the bad guy in all this. I did ask my therapist how we could all get in the right mindset, and this is what he had to offer," I added.

HOW TO GET IN THE RIGHT MINDSET

"So, now we know 'what' we need to do, but someone is going to need to tell me how. You girls know me, I need step-by-step instructions," Robbie stated.

"Don't even worry, I got you covered. The therapist gave me an entire list of ways to get in the game, so to speak," I concluded.

Here are some of the tips to get into the right mindset for strength training that he offered:

- **Set clear goals:** Prior to initiating any strength training regimen, establish specific objectives regarding what you intend to accomplish. Doing this can help you stay motivated and be able to focus throughout your workout. If you want to lose weight, strengthen your muscles, or tone overall, state your goal clearly.

- **Visualize success:** Take a few moments to visualize yourself successfully completing your workout and reaching your goals. Such a practice can enhance your confidence and motivation.
- **Listen to music:** Incorporating music into your workout routine can assist in achieving a positive mindset and overcoming physical challenges. Choose music with a strong beat and motivational lyrics.
- **Warm up properly:** Take the time to warm up your muscles before you start your strength training. Starting with a warm-up session can diminish the chances of injury and prepare your body for the upcoming workout.
- **Focus on form:** Maintaining proper form while using weights is crucial as it can help you optimize the effectiveness of your workout and minimize the chances of injury.
- **Stay positive:** A positive mindset can be highly beneficial in strength training. Shifting your focus from your limitations to your strengths and celebrating your progress as you move forward can be more effective than fixating on what you cannot do.

"Okay, this guy seems to know his shit. I already feel better equipped to start this strength training journey. Thank you, Franny, for meeting with him and getting us this great information," Robbie speaks up.

"It was my pleasure. I wanted to ensure we all had a great start to this. Looking ahead, I immediately thought motivation would be what gets our butts moving," I said in conclusion.

4

WE NEED A TRAINER!

A fter our weekend together and our critically important chat regarding our health, the tribe knows what needs to be done. First, we must meet with a trainer to address our health issues. We leave the decision to find the best trainer for our needs in Nora's capable hands. She has our medical records and will make us an appointment asap.

Please note that it is optional but always feasible for everyone to do this. Some fantastic gyms offer a personal trainer, free for your first two visits. Make the most of this service and utilize the time to ask targeted questions that cater to your needs. If you fall in any of the same categories the tribe is dealing with, you should have a comprehensive knowledge base at the end of this book, but feel free to dive deeper with your physician before meeting with your trainer.

If you need help finding a gym that offers this, *YouTube* has impressive tutorial videos, and I will supply the link to some at the end of this book in a resource section. But, again, always check with your physician before beginning any new routine.

For the next four weeks, Nora will stay in her new condo, and Robbie will work from her laptop in Arizona as she stays with me, so the tribe can kick-start this health journey together and have each other for support.

THE MEET AND GREET

Today is the big day! The tribe sisters will meet their strength and conditioning coach Marco for the first time, and he will tell us what he has laid out for each of us in terms of a plan.

Welcome Marco

Last night was an emotional roller-coaster for us ladies, but we enthusiastically greet our new trainer today. After an indulgent breakfast—as we feel it may be our last—we fling the doors of that gym open with the vigor of women half our age. Now, I want to make one thing clear. I, Franny Russo, am already spritzing the air with my body spray because I cannot decipher that mix of smells punishing my nostrils. Rotting gym socks with a hint of pain and suffering, perhaps? Focus, Franny, focus!

It is then that I hear Nora's shaky voice, "Stop it this instant, is that him?" I sense the flirtatious nature in her tone as I slowly turn around to witness what can only be described as if Denzel Washington and The Rock had a baby.

"Good afternoon, ladies, I am Marco, and I am delighted to meet your acquaintance," he says, reaching out to shake our hands. Oh, did I mention he was wearing a suit? Mop me up off the floor. At this time, Robbie leans in to remind me I have a son older than him, which snaps me back to reality.

"If I could please escort you all to my office, we have plenty to cover today," he asks. We all follow Marco into a well-organized space containing models of joints of the body and books everywhere. "If you don't mind, I would like to give you a run down of who I am and why I am passionate about this profession to begin with."

"Please do," Nora nods in his direction.

"First I would like to thank you for coming down and visiting with me today. I always like to begin these sessions by explaining to clients what my job title means to me, what it is I do, and why I am personally passionate about it," Marco explains.

"I believe I have two jobs with each client—to strengthen their muscles and to reduce their chance of injury. I always like to ask myself *what makes a strengthening coach*, so I know I am offering my clients all they need. From me, you can also expect the following:

- An individualized plan to meet your specific needs.
- Be your personal moral leader for your group.
- I will always come to each session prepared.
- To effectively communicate to you and make space for you to be heard.
- As a certified nutritionist, I can give advice in this area as well.
- Act as a liaison between you and your healthcare team with any medical updates.
- The best motivator you need on those tough days.
- Explain each and every exercise we do and how it will help you specifically."

Marco explains that having a strength and conditioning coach with excellent skill and technique is one thing, but if they fall flat on customer experience, you will not continue your health journey.

"Any questions so far ladies?" Marco politely asks.

Robbie is the first to throw her arm into the air, and I am convinced she will ask if there is a smoothie bar on the premises because I have heard her stomach growl four times. "Marco, clear something up for me, please. What exactly is strength training because I don't want to be looking like Arnold Schwarzenegger out here," she says, curling her bicep.

"Great question Robbie," he answers before busting out into his definition.

There are a lot of terms that people use interchangeably: strength training, weight training, and resistance exercise. We are strength training, which is the umbrella term covering all the other ones. Strength training relates to activities that use any resistance to strengthen your muscles. It is that resistance that makes the skeletal muscles contract. We can create resistance using various weight machines, resistance bands, dumbbells, or our body weight (Eustice, 2023).

"Thank you for clearing that up for me," Robbie chimes in.

"It is my job and passion to see each client through from start to finish," Marco explains. "This career chose me after losing both parents to debilitating diseases that I believe could have been prevented from healthier choices. I wake up each day passionate to give knowledge to those who want to live a long and healthy life," he says with everything we need to hear.

Nora pops up off her chair with enough enthusiasm for this entire tribe, "Marco you are an inspiring human, and I want to speak on behalf of all of us when I say thank you for taking this task on."

We all stand and shake his hand, asking, when do we get started?

"Right now," he beams as he grabs his notebooks and visitor badges.

I am the first to protest, and I make all the excuses, from us not having the right gear to us eating a huge breakfast. Robbie giggles and farts.

Robbie says, laughing, "See, Marco, I am too gassy for this today!"

He reassures us this is simply an intake session and a tour. I exhale with the force of a beluga whale. We set out to examine the guts of the beast, as I like to call it. Marco points at machines and mats as if it were his own personal castle, and Nora nods as though acknowledging she used it just yesterday. Robbie and I, locking arms for security, are sweating and out of breath, just trying to keep up.

"I am convinced I already have a thigh rash just from this tour," Robbie whispers through laughter. "But seriously, do we have to do wind sprints just to see it all," she continues. At this time, I beg her to stop so I don't pee myself before this wraps up. We finally circle back to Marco's office before my allergy to workout gear flares up, and he asks Robbie and me if we are okay as he notices our laborious breathing.

"Oh sweet Marco, this is why we are here, *this* is our normal!" I spout out, still trying to catch my breath.

"Okay ladies, if you don't mind, I would just like to review your individual plans with you now," Marco states eagerly.

My Strengthening Plan for Pre-surgery

"Franny, the beginning stages of your plan will focus on strengthening your muscles to prepare for your hip replacement surgery. We will often reduce our mobility quite a lot before this type of surgery because the cartilage in the joint is gone, meaning any movement within it is very painful. In addition, due to the lack of activity and exercise, the muscles are now relatively weak.

Unfortunately, this can mean a longer recovery time. So, our goal is to get those muscles stronger before surgery so the recovery is shorter and less painful," Marco explained. (Allina Health's Public Health Department, 2000).

Marco's goal is to meet with me 30 minutes daily, five days a week. He will get me started on exercises to build muscle correctly with instructions on how to do them at home those first two weeks before returning to the gym. He highlights multiple times that the exercises will cease immediately if the pain is ever felt, and I am to rest for 10 minutes before trying again.

Below are the eight strengthening exercises Marco assigned to me to begin before hip replacement surgery (Allina Health's Public Health Department, 2000):

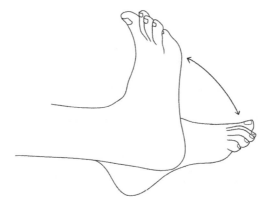

• **Ankle Pumps:** With your legs straight out in front of you, pull your feet up toward you—toes pointing to the sky—now push your toes down toward the floor. Hold each for a count of five. Three repetitions are ideal.

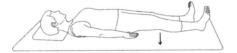

• **Thigh Squeezes:** Laying flat on your back, push the back of your kneecap down. You should feel a tightening in the top of your thigh muscle. Hold for five and relax. Five repetitions are ideal.

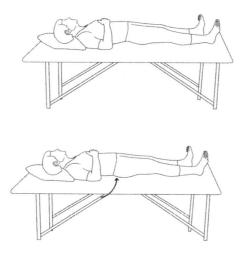

• **Glute Squeezes:** Laying flat on your back, squeeze your buttocks together, hold for five, and release. Five repetitions are best.

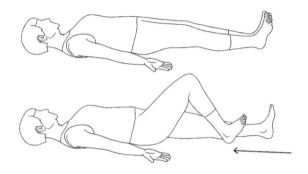

• **Heel Slides:** Laying flat on your back, support your head with a pillow. Bend the knee on the side of your body where you will have surgery. Using your heel to slide, slide your heel up as far as you can comfortably toward your buttocks and then back down. Five repetitions are ideal.

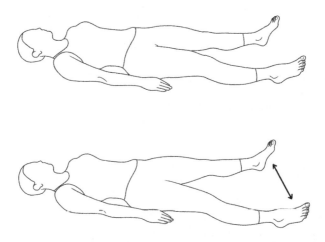

• **Hip Abductions:** Flat on your back once again, you will slide your surgical leg out to the side as far out to the side—without feeling pain—while keeping your leg straight and your knee always pointing up. Ten repetitions are best.

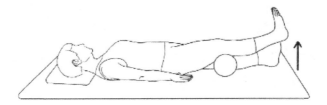

• **Lying Kicks:** Still on your back, place a foam roller under the knee of your surgical leg. Straighten that surgical leg while that foam roller is under the knee. Hold that position for 10 seconds. Lower your leg and rest for ten, and repeat. Ten repetitions are ideal.

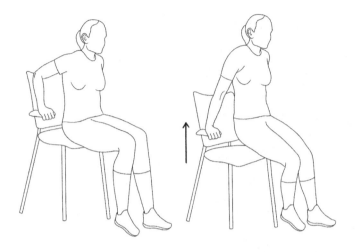

- **Chair Pushup:** This exercise requires a sturdy chair with arms. While holding the arms of the chair, push down on the arms and straighten your elbows, raising your butt just a few inches off the seat. The goal here is to work up to holding yourself up longer and longer each time. Start with a count of five and continue to build.

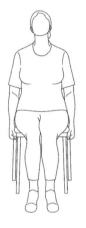 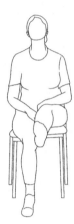

- **Sitting Kick:** Sitting on that same sturdy chair, straighten the knee of your surgical leg. Start by trying to hold it for five seconds. Your goal is to hold it for longer each time.

The above exercises are designed to build the muscles in both my legs, but dominantly the leg on the surgical side. This strengthening will help ease the pain and speed up my recovery after hip replacement surgery. However, not wanting to overwhelm me all at once, Marco decides to wait and discuss my post-surgical plan later.

"Wow, Marco, I have to say, this doesn't terrify me because in my mind, I was picturing vertical jumps and hurdles," I remarked as I reviewed my plan. Marco snickers as he reassures me that, in due time, he will have me loving his world as much as he does.

Nora's Strengthening Plan

Nora's strengthening plan will focus on maintaining her current workout regime by adjusting her training to accommodate her as she ages. Nora loves to be physically active but has noticed her muscles becoming sorer and needing more time to recover. In addition, as we age, our muscles become more elastic and can be damaged easier, so giving Nora exercises she can do without that fear is vital.

Marco quickly points out to all the ladies that strength training slows down the aging process (Freytag, 2022).

"Wait, what did you just say?" I asked Marco with surprise.

"It is true and well-researched that all exercise, but mainly strength training, is the best anti-aging remedy around!" Marco boasts, now gaining all of the sister tribe's attention.

Marco knows Nora struggles to adapt to her exercise routine, aging, and mental health. So, why exactly does Nora need to make these changes now (Freytag, 2022):

- **Strength training to build lean muscle for women over 50:** Nora loves to burn calories by doing cardio, which is great for her overall heart health, but when that fat melts away, those muscles need to be strengthened as we age. Being strong as we age gives us the freedom to be independent longer. By the age of 40, we, as women, start to lose muscle mass if we do nothing to replace it.
- **Strength training to build bone density for women over 50:** We need to know that falls are the leading cause of injury, hospitalization, and even death in women over 50. Strength training builds muscle and reinforces the connective tissues that surround your bones. This training makes you, as a whole, stronger and prevents those falls in the first place.
- **Speeding up women's metabolism with strength training:** As we age, our metabolism slows down, but strength training can kick it back into gear. Yes, you heard that right. A resting metabolic rate (RMR) is calculated by how many calories your body burns while resting. The fact is, the more muscle you have, the higher your RMR will be. To break that down even further, the more muscles you have, the more calories you burn daily.

- **Our mental health will improve with strength training:** I cannot say this clearly enough. Aging is not easy, and this is not for all the reasons most people assume. Women are expected to give up most of their identity as a mother and their careers and then are asked to knit and bake cookies the second a grandchild appears on the scene. We are looked at as "acting out" if we choose to explore the world or invest in ourselves, we are expected to act our age and slide into senior living, sensible shoes and polyester in hand. This mindset tanks our mental health faster than most can understand. Depression, anxiety, loss of self, and lack of confidence begin to build. Investing in physical health by adopting a strength training program has been proven to boost our confidence and mental health immediately.

- **Strength training for women improves balance and mobility:** As we age, there are no longer rules that say we can't enroll in a yoga or belly dancing class. But, if our body says, "Girl, what the hell are we doing," you may need to rethink your bucket list. A strength training program will improve your balance, coordination, and mobility, allowing you to pluck things off that list you have always wanted to do. Want to take a salsa dancing class? Please do it! Want to celebrate your 60th birthday by jumping out of a plane? Please do it!

Marco wanted to assemble a set of strength exercises for Nora to work out all her muscle groups. These particular exercises are designed to use Nora's body weight instead of weights, so Nora can learn to power down her workouts as she moves into her 60s and 70s. Nora needs to learn to listen to her body, and on the days she is in pain, she would alter her workouts to use no weights and allow her body weight to be enough. On days she feels great and can use weights to assist her.

Instructions: Each exercise should be attempted for 10 to 12 repetitions, and complete each round of exercises in full, twice.

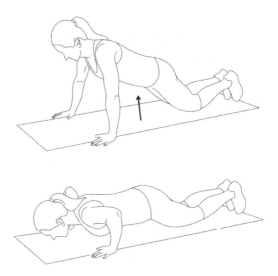

Modified Push Ups

1. You will want to start in a kneeling position, hands below your shoulders and knees behind your hips.
2. You should be staring straight in front of your fingertips so your neck is stretched long. Keep your butt cheeks and inner thighs squeezed tight together.
3. Lower yourself slowly to the ground while keeping your elbows at a 45-degree angle.
4. Push yourself back to the starting position.
5. Repeat this for the required repetitions.

Muscles Targeted: This exercise targets the following muscles; the chest, upper body, back, shoulders, biceps and triceps, and the core (Freytag, 2022).

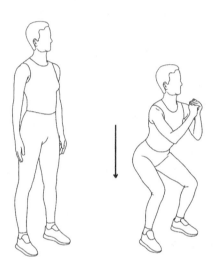

Basic Squat

1. Keep your feet hip-width apart and your back nice and straight while standing. Remember that your hips, toes, and knees point straight ahead.
2. Now, bend your knees and sit as if you are going to sit down in a chair. Again, keeping your weight distributed equally on both heels is

essential, allowing you to keep your knees behind your toes.

3. Get to the bottom of your squat, pause for a moment, and then slowly rise back up to a full standing position. Repeat the whole movement for the required repetitions.

Muscles Targeted: This exercise targets the following muscles; the glutes, quads, hamstrings, and core (Freytag, 2022).

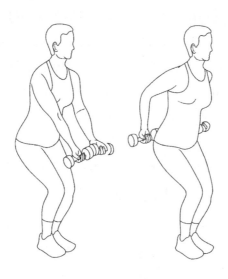

Reverse Grip Double Arm Row

1. To start this exercise, position your feet together and lean forward slightly into a squat. This movement engages your abdominal muscles and glutes. Hold a pair of two-pound hand weights with your palms facing upward and your arms stretched out in front of your body.
2. Bring your elbows back by squeezing your upper back muscles together and pull the elbows gently past your hips. You should feel your lats—the muscle just under your shoulder blades—and your triceps—located on the back of your upper arm—engage, then return to the starting position.

Muscle Groups Targeted: This exercise targets the upper body, shoulders, back, and triceps (Freytag, 2022).

Marco intentionally only gave Nora three exercises to start because they discussed adapting her current routine by lowering the amount of weight she uses. He also suggests giving her mental health an immediate boost by doing these exercises outdoors as often as possible.

Because Nora is coming from the Midwest and into a climate that permits more Vitamin D, he wants to tackle any symptoms of seasonal affective disorder (SAD). This occurs in some people who live in environments that see longer hours of darkness in colder winter months. As a result, their serotonin production slows down, which then causes their melatonin to be all out of whack. All of this generates our sleep patterns to become a mess, and depression can also sneak its way in (HealthMatch, 2022). By suggesting Nora do a portion of her strengthening exercises outdoors in that sunshine, vitamin D will seep in through her pores and boost the production of serotonin naturally.

As much as Nora snickered and scoffed throughout her plan's presentation, Marco reassures her at the end that he can tell by the shape of her body and the report from her doctor that she is more than capable of the plan he has presented to her. "Nora, I don't want to discourage you by what I have put in front of you," Marco begins. "My intention is to put you on a path of learning what strengthening exercises you can learn that won't injure your muscles as you progress into this next chapter," he explains.

Nora must understand that if she continues on her path, she will do permanent damage to herself that could require surgery or joint replacement in the near future. Unfortunately, Nora only understands one speed in her life—fast and perfect. This is Marco's attempt to show her a safe and pain-free way to allow her changing body to stay healthy and in shape.

"Marco, this adjustment I have to make is of no reflection of your knowledge and hard work," Nora starts. "I have work to do that includes acceptance of where I am in this next phase of life, but I will do what is needed, and I truly love the outdoor component of this." Nora snatches up the papers and gives a smile.

Robbie's Strengthening Plan

Marco is aware that the strengthening plan for Robbie needs to be centered around her recent diagnosis of osteoarthritis and having to reduce weight. However, he knows this will be a challenging plan to execute, as those with osteoarthritis are always in pain, so convincing them to move can be tricky.

Marco turns his attention to Robbie, kindness filling his eyes as he begins to speak. "I understand that this condition—osteoarthritis—is unbelievably painful, so I want to tell you that I honor your bravery in fighting through this." I see Robbie brush a tear from her cheek as she motions for Marco to carry on.

When it comes to osteoarthritis, Marco recommends range-of-motion and low-impact exercises. He will work up to strength training as the pain allows. He will work hand in hand with Robbie's healthcare team so her pain stays at bay, allowing them to add weight, build that muscle, and take the load off her joints. This will take some time as they have to be extremely careful. The last thing they want to do is injure any of the joints.

"If at any time you experience pain in a joint, we will scale back on the amount of weight we are using, or return to no weight at all."

Studies are now showing us that without strength training, by the time we are 80, our muscle mass is 50% of what it was when we were just 30 years old (Eustice, 2023). It drops that quickly. If we do nothing to replace that muscle, we set ourselves up for mobility, coordination, and injury issues.

Below, I have created an essential list of things for you to remember regarding your specific needs and requirements (Eustice, 2023):

- Never apply pain analgesics before working out. They may mask pain during exercise, and we never want to work past a pain spot and risk injury. You are free to use them after.
- When doing any of the exercises we learn together at home, be sure to stretch lightly

before beginning. Our joints need that prior to starting.

- With osteoarthritis, we tend to want to work on the side that doesn't cause pain. This will cause us to become unbalanced in our muscle strength, so you must work both sides of the body evenly to avoid this.
- Use ice packs to decrease inflammation after your workout.
- Use a hot pack on your affected joints before a workout to increase circulation.
- Hydrate, hydrate, hydrate!

Now we know that despite osteoarthritis being painful, we still need to move those joints. Moving them brings oxygen, blood flow, and nutrients into the cartilage. We want and need this because it will allow those joints to last as long as you (Liao, 2017)!

Marco put together three strengthening exercises for Robbie that use no weights, to begin with first.

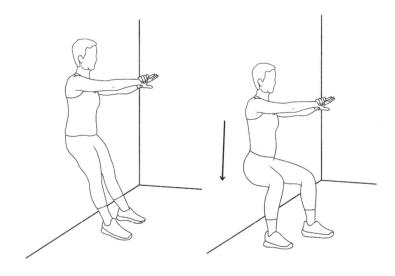

Mini Wall Squats

To begin, stand and place your head and back against a wall. Be sure your feet are shoulder-width apart. Now, squat down with your knees bent at a 30-degree angle. Slowly stand back up, keeping your butt, and thighs squeezed tight. Repeat eight times. To add shoulder resistance, put your arms straight out in front of you while doing this exercise (Liao, 2017).

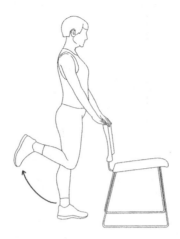

One Leg Balance

Start by standing next to a table or a solid surface, then place one hand on it to support yourself. Now, you should lift one leg while you balance on the other foot for a maximum of 10 seconds. After that, you can use one finger or completely relinquish your support as you gain strength and confidence. Now, switch to the other side so you are working the muscles on both sides of your body. The end goal will be to fully support yourself, allowing your core muscles to do the work (Liao, 2017).

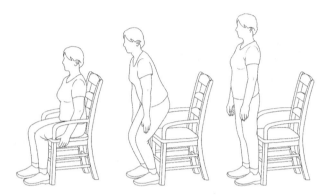

Sit To Stand

For this exercise, you should choose a sturdy chair with arms. Sit firmly in the chair. Now, slowly and intentionally, raise yourself to your feet. Be sure to clench your butt and thigh muscles together while doing so. Next, lower yourself back down to a seated position, being mindful to keep those muscles tight. Do not use your arms to assist you during this exercise. If you have joint pain, use the armrests to help you. Repeat 15 times (Liao, 2017).

Range of Motion Exercises

These exercises are intended to get those stiff and achy joints loosened up and moving more freely without the pain. It is ideal to work these into your workout routine three times per week to begin.

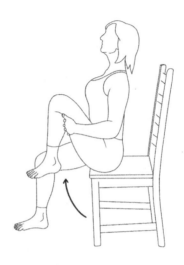

Sitting Knee Flexion

To begin this workout, you will need a sturdy chair that won't roll or flip. Now, you will want to sit just on the edge of it. Next, lift one of your knees, putting your shin in your hands. With ease, pull your chin in toward your thigh. Hold this position for three seconds, then lower your leg back down. Next, move to the other leg and repeat ten times (Liao, 2017).

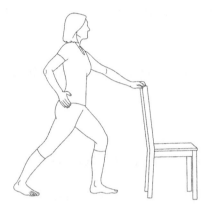

Standing Hip Flexor Stretch

For this exercise, I want you to step one foot forward, forcing your feet to be hip-distance apart. Now, go ahead and bend that back leg just a touch, and slowly bend your front knee while keeping your upper body nice and straight. Hold this position for 10 seconds and repeat it ten times. Hold onto the wall if you need additional support (Liao, 2017).

Robbie takes this all in, and a smile comes across her face. "Marco, I cannot guarantee I won't fart or pee just a bit during some of these, but I will show up, and I will bust my ass," she says with a look of determination on her face.

"Ladies, I am so proud of the three of you because working through pain is the most courageous work we can do," Marco remarks as he moves us toward the door.

We all shake hands and tell him we will see him first thing next week.

HOW ARE WE GOING TO DO THIS?

"Alright ladies, let's head to lunch and discuss all we just had dumped in our laps. What do you say?" Robbie says from the backseat.

I pull up to one of our favorite local margarita bars, and we quickly convene in our "spot" on the patio. Honestly, the group is tough to read now, so I do what I always do in tense situations—order a pitcher of dirty margaritas!

Nora is the first to begin the conversation, and I am shocked to hear her response. "If Marco thinks I am about to abandon the workout I have been using for 20 years for one that has me acting like I am 80, he is out of his mind."

Robbie quickly follows suit. "Did you hear him say how he 'understood' my pain, is he serious? He is lucky I didn't throat punch him at that moment and I'm serious, I am going to be one huge gas bag through all of that crap!"

I quickly determined the girls needed a pep talk: "Girls, I am as excited as a dental hygienist on denture cleaning day. Okay, but we need to do this. What is our alternative? Look at us right now—you have the friend who dunks double-stuffed Oreos in her wine being your cheerleader. The one who has never placed lycra on her ass a day in her life? How is this at all right?"

How to Avoid Muscle Cramps

On the top of Marco's list is staying hydrated. I am going to need a lot of reminders on this topic because we all know how much I hate drinking water. I get it, though. If it will help me avoid those charley horses, count me in. I added the tips Marco gave us below:

- Stay hydrated: Just as Marco says, dehydration is your main cause of muscle cramps. By ensuring you are drinking plenty of water before, during, and after your workout, you are making sure your muscles have enough fluid to function correctly.
- Warm-up: Warm up all your muscle groups before you begin your strength training routine. You can do this with some light cardio and deep stretching. This not only helps

prevent cramping, but it also increases your range of motion.

- Stretching: Regular stretching, especially after your workout, will aid in the prevention of muscle cramps. Remember to stretch the muscle groups you worked on during your weight training session.
- Nutrition: If you are low on electrolytes, sodium, magnesium, or potassium, you need to make sure you up your intake through nutrition and supplements. These key minerals aid in the regulation of muscle contractions and prevent cramps.
- Proper form: You need to be using proper form when doing strength training exercises to help you prevent cramping. If you focus on keeping your good posture and avoid overexerting your muscles, you will help eliminate cramping.
- Rest and recovery: Ensuring you get the proper amount of rest and recovery time between workouts is critical for preventing muscle cramps. If you overtrain, this can lead to muscle fatigue, and this increases the risk of cramping.

"Well, I will cheer for that advice. So far, nothing I don't feel I can stick to," Robbie says, raising her margarita glass. "Wasn't Marco trying to emphasize stretching for more than muscle cramps?" Nora asked.

Make Sure You Stretch

"Oh, how right you are, Nora. Marco couldn't say enough about stretching and warming up before we work out. He elaborated extensively on the importance of preparing the body for exercise," I stated. Below, I added some of the reasons Marco says stretching is necessary."

- Preventing injuries: How does stretching and warming up help to reduce the risk of injury during physical activity? Great question. When you do this, it prepares your muscles, joints, and tendons for strength training. The last thing you want to be doing is jumping in with both feet and cold muscles. Take the time to warm up.
- Increasing your flexibility: When we stretch before beginning our workout, it helps to improve our flexibility. This is important because it can increase your range of motion as well as improve your overall performance during exercise.
- Improving your circulation: If you take the time to warm up, you increase the blood flow to

your muscles. Why is this important? Because that blood flow is how oxygen and nutrients are delivered to your muscles and get them ready for physical activity.

- Enhancing your performance: When you warm up and stretch, you can help to enhance your physical performance by improving your flexibility, mobility, and range of motion.
- Reduced soreness: Stretching after exercise is important because it can help to reduce those sore muscles and stiffness. This can happen as a result of exercise-induced muscle damage.
- Mental preparation: We all know that committing to strength training requires motivation and mental toughness. Stretching and warming up will help you mentally prepare for exercise by reducing stress and increasing your focus.

"Marco was amazing at supplying us with this information because it will ensure we get the best out of our strength training," Nora chimes in. "Love the guy, but I am all tapped out on Marco today and am ready to go shopping for our gear," Robbie says, getting up from her chair.

It truly has been a long and mentally exhausting day, hasn't it? However, now that I am stuffed with great food and drinks, I do believe we have earned that shopping spree!

LET'S GO SHOPPING

Our tribe loves to shop, but we all have niches we enjoy shopping for. Nora is our group's book and baby shopper, especially since becoming a grandmother. She also cannot pass up a new pair of tights because, as we mentioned, she is always in workout gear.

Robbie squeals in delight over new pajamas, fuzzy blankets, slippers, and all things that comfort her or those she loves. I always state that her favorite sense is touch; she can't walk through a store without touching everything.

I am told I must have been a magpie in my previous life because I love all things shiny and colorful. If it catches my eye, all rationale goes out the window. I have shown up at my relatively small condo with a rather large art piece without knowing where or if it would fit in any location because it was visually appealing, and I had to have it.

I can assure you only one of us in the tribe sister's group enjoys shopping for clothing, and she is dragging us kicking and screaming today.

"Good morning girls, I hope you all slept well because today is going to be a great day!" Nora says, with the enthusiasm of the head cheerleader. Me, eyes barely open and demanding coffee, places my finger against my pursed lips, gesturing for Nora to quiet down just a bit. "Nora, what freaking time is it? Is the sun even up yet?" Robbie asks, the sleep mask still firmly in place.

"I have a full day planned, and breakfast is on the table," Nora barks, heading into the kitchen. "The early bird gets all the sales, and the car will leave in one hour!" I throw my pillow at her as she leaves my room.

We arrive at some mall that Nora claims have all the "best" stores for the workout wear we need. On the way there, Robbie and I clarified that we would not be stepping foot in any store that didn't serve our size. We will not be humiliated by any salesperson convincing us to "just try it on" only to be dripping in sweat, stuck in a sports bra, fearing the only way out is a pair of scissors.

"I want comfort and breathability because there will be plenty of bending and even more sweating, got it?" Robbie blurts out as we make our way into the mall.

Six hours—six damn hours, people, and we all left with enough workout gear to get started on this journey. I am convinced I pulled four muscles, farted twice, peed a bit, and sweat enough to consider this as two full workout days.

"I have two questions," Robbie asks, raising her hand from the backseat and chugging her second bottle of water. "First, why in the actual hell do they feel the need to make store temperatures a million degrees at all times? Second, did they always have funhouse mirrors in changing rooms, or is this new?" she asks with a grave expression on her face.

Nora laughed so hard that her drinking water came straight from her nose. I clap my hands in solidarity with Robbie. I crank the air conditioning to ease our overheated core temperatures.

"Well, I consider this a victory," Nora states, a massive smile on her face. She isn't wrong. Despite all of our bitching and moaning, we all have a great wardrobe to begin our strength training workouts.

Women, as we age, can struggle with how to dress. When it comes to workout gear, this world can be intimidating. I have listed some helpful tips below to make that shopping journey easier for you, the reader (Roussy, 2022).

- **Tops:** You want your workout clothing to be comfortable. Cotton t-shirts can be worn, but they aren't known for being super breathable, and when they get soaked in sweat, they don't allow you to move easily. Workout tops can be a t-shirt, a tank top, or possibly a thin, long sleeve shirt. It is your choice; it depends on how hot you run, your activity, and your comfort level.

- **Bottoms:** There is no shortage of workout bottoms to pick from. Whether you select crops, shorts, leggings, or pants, keep in mind comfort is vital. Always remember to keep the type of workout you are doing in mind. If anyone mentions your age should impact your choice in wearing workout leggings, walk away. Those comments are ageist; you don't need to waste time or energy addressing them.

- **Bras:** Hear this! Your bra is the most essential piece in your workout clothing arsenal. A sports bra must support you, especially for running or high-impact workouts. Supporting your beautiful breasts with a perfectly-fitted bra will make you feel better while you work out. I recommend avoiding sports bras that slide over your head. They can be challenging to put on and uncomfortable. However, I do recommend finding those with a front closure.

- **Jackets:** These are just a good idea to have for a few reasons. Whether you are just taking a nice walk around your neighborhood or using them to arrive or leave the gym. Try to choose one that is lightweight and moisture-wicking to keep you dry.

- **Shoes:** Another essential aspect of your workout gear that you want to pay much attention to. Your shoes need to fit you well, offer excellent ankle support and do the job you need them to. If you are a runner, be sure that is the purpose of your shoe. If you need them to help with balance, mention that to your salesperson. The sole should have a good grip but not be so thick that it could be a tripping concern. Comfort and breathability are key here.

Tomorrow is the big day as the tribe will be starting their strength training program. The tribe has had a busy time meeting with their trainer and making time to gather all they need to get started. Follow along to find out what time of day is best to work out and why you should trust your body's signals and your trainer.

5

I WILL PICK YOU UP AT 8!

The tribe sisters have endured medical appointments, met with their new trainer Marco, and survived the mall while shopping for workout gear. Now, the day has arrived. Robbie made a fantastic meal last night for the women, and Nora gave her pep talk before they all hit the sack at a decent time.

"I will come and pick you both up at 8:00 a.m.," Nora says just before leaving to head back to her condo for the evening.

THE HELL YOU WILL!

Robbie slowly lowers her glass of wine, and with just a look, Nora knows the tribe is unhappy about the morning pickup time. "Ladies listen, I am well aware how much you hate waking up early, so I went ahead and did some research."

- **Don't work out after dinner:** This option may be appealing because we can have more time during these hours, but it can mess up our sleep schedules. Sleep is critical and necessary for our overall health as we age, and we should avoid anything that can disrupt it. For example, *"Sports Medicine"* published 23 studies, finding that a workout just an hour before sleep can cause insomnia and lower overall sleep quality (Stutz et al., 2018).

- **Working out close to bedtime causes issues:** Sleep issues become an issue as we age. Our aging brain needs that whole night's rest to refuel. Our body counts on that rest; without it, we can have long-term issues such as memory deterioration, risk of stroke, high blood pressure, and heart disease (Anderer, 2021). One other statistic that is important to understand is that sleep deprivation is one thing that can age us faster than most things. They published a study in *Brain, Behavior, and Immunity* that found one night of poor sleep activated genes associated with aging (Carroll et al., 2016).

- **Why early morning workouts are beneficial:**
  We must know that cognitive decline is
  expected as we get older. However, the British
  Journal of Sports Medicine has shown that
  morning workouts will improve our cognition
  and mental sharpness (Wheeler et al., 2019).

"Nora, how long did you take to prepare that presentation?" Robbie asks, knowing our workout pickup times will start bright and early. Nora gives us her best smile and wave as she heads out the door.

AM I SUPPOSED TO PEE AND FART?

The tribe rolled up to the gym, exited the vehicle, flinging our bags over our shoulders, and entered our new hangout place as if it was the first day of high school. Hair on point, new outfits, brand new shoes, and excitement for our new adventure. As long as we were together, we could do anything.

When I looked up, I caught a glimpse of Marco waiting to greet us at the door. He snapped a photo of us, mentioning how he likes to use these before photos as inspiration.

Once dressed in our gear, Marco prepares us for our 45-minute workout. With each of us at our own station, Nora is working on core strength, for Robbie, it is leg day, and I will be focusing on my hips—preparing for surgery.

After Marco has Nora all set up, he leaves her to it, knowing she has a good knowledge base. He makes his way over to Robbie, who is lying flat on her back on the yoga mat, ready for a mid-morning nap. Within three seconds, I hear the familiar sound of her "embarrassed giggle," followed by her repeated apology.

"Marco I am *so* sorry, but I tried to warn you that you were in the line of fire." Robbie says through her continued laughter. With her face still flaming red, I decipher that she farted right in his face the second he used his body weight to force her knee toward her body.

As he makes his way over to me, I feel a sense of panic. "Listen, Marco, I saw what happened over there on the mat, and I am making no promises," I state with a smirk. Marco is fully aware that I need to focus on strengthening the muscles and joints around my hips before surgery. Today, he wants me to concentrate on "chair sits." As he has me sit in a sturdy chair, I immediately think what a cakewalk my first day is. Listening to his explicit instructions, I firmly clench my butt, thighs, and core as I raise myself slowly from the chair. He instructed me on how to keep my spine aligned.

STRENGTH TRAINING FOR WOMEN OVER 50 | 99

"Imagine you have a string coming out the top of your head, and I am pulling you straight up from the ceiling," he remarked, gesturing at what this might look like. He reminded me to keep everything tight as I lowered myself back down. It was the fifth repetition when it happened. As I raised my ass off that seat, I sneezed, farted, and pissed myself simultaneously. The aging woman's trifecta! Okay, it was more like a dribbling of sorts, but my granny panties were damp, and my dignity was in the toilet where the urine should have been.

Marco did what any gentleman would do and acted like he heard and saw nothing. He excused himself, pretending to take a call. Mortified, I sat on that chair, motioning for Nora. "What's wrong? You have that same expression as the day you shit your pants on the roller-coaster in tenth grade—did you shit yourself?" Nora asks, eyes wide, waiting for my answer.

"This dumb-ass strength training made me piss my pants and fart right in Marco's face. Now I am sitting here in my pissy granny panties, and all I want to do is go home." I say, feeling defeated. Nora loops her arm under mine and marches my sorry pissy ass to the changing room. Robbie, noticing the commotion, quickly follows suit. Nora orders me into the shower but soon realizes who she is talking to.

Franny Russo would never be caught dead using a public shower. I stomp into the bathroom stall with my bag, change out of my wet panties and emerge victorious. "Girls, how am I supposed to face that man now?" I ask, looking for an honest answer.

Robbie, the first to pipe up, informs me that she farted *loudly* in his face five minutes after we arrived. "Not only that, Franny, but it also smelled exactly like that hard-boiled egg I ate in the car on the way here."

Marco texted me on my phone, asking if he could speak with us in his office.

"Before any of you ladies say a word, I need all three of you to understand that I, in my 10 years as a personal trainer,:

- I have been thrown up on
- I have been pooped on
- I have been bled on
- I have performed CPR 11 times
- I have been farted on too many times to remember
- I have farted over a dozen times in a client's face
- I have been peed on
- I have been sworn at
- I have been laughed at

- I have been a shoulder to cry on."

Marco continues to tell us that there is little he hasn't seen, heard, or experienced in this role.

"You ladies must understand that flatulence, urinating, and yes, even pooping are all a normal part of the human body and when we start bending and twisting, those fluids and air are given an escape route." he explains.

Marco is bang on here. Strength training, in particular, is one group of exercises that produces the most gas. While training, we are instructed to squeeze and tighten our core muscles as we lift our bodies or weights. Unfortunately, when we do this, our digestive tract does the same. As a result, air often gets trapped, and if we forget to breathe and exhale, farting is imminent (Kassel, 2022).

"I love the medical explanation," Nora pipes up. "But can we give the girls some insight into what they are shoveling into their faces before coming here and how that plays into all this as well?"

Marco continues on with his gassy lesson, informing us that if we choose a morning workout, we should avoid high-fiber breakfast foods. Doing this can help our gut and "fart anxiety," as he calls it.

Some foods to avoid in the morning would be (Kassel, 2022):

- beans
- dairy
- fruit
- onions
- sugar
- carbonated drinks

"Indulge all you want once you wrap up your workout, but to avoid that gassy, bloated feeling, refrain from them for breakfast," Marco instructs.

I stand up, my dignity somewhat back in check, and reach to shake Marco's hand. "It is okay, sir; I have washed up," I joked.

I thank Marco for this enlightening information and for being so gracious. Typically, this would have been enough for me to storm out to my car, mumbling *I told you so*, and never return again.

Before letting us leave, Marco reminds us of our "homework."

"Huh, I know I did not sign off on that," Robbie says, still wiping the sweat from her face.

"Did you all read your welcome packets?" Nora asks, bragging rights written all over her smug mug.

Marco reminds us that within our welcome packet, there is a note stating that each Monday, there will be a brief summary of what our week will entail, a few do's and don'ts, and a few recipes to try.

Nora stated, "We will see you in the morning, Marco! I am dragging this tribe out of here before they eat you for lunch."

DON'T FORGET TO BREATHE!

I first stumbled upon an article on four mistakes we must avoid when lifting weights and strength training. I feel this odd twinge in my gut. I can't stop staring at the woman's face on the front page of this article. I don't yet know if it is the sheer determination in her eyes or if I can suddenly see myself in her. Is this excitement I'm feeling? Holy shit, I think it is!

The article begins.

"Regardless of gender or age, if you decide to start lifting weights, you will lower your body fat, increase your resting heart rate, improve your balance and motor coordination, and improve your joint stability" (Cleveland Clinic, 2016).

You should aim for 20 to 30 minutes of working out three days a week to achieve these incredible results. The same goes for lifting weights; it is recommended for a total body workout of 20 to 30 minutes three days a week (Cleveland Clinic, 2020).

Be mindful that it is easy to make mistakes that could cause injuries. Let's discuss the most common mistakes to steer clear of while you're lifting weights during your strength training. They are as follows (Cleveland Clinic, 2020):

- **Don't hold your breath:** How often do you recall bending over to lift a heavy piece of furniture, then holding your breath as you lift? We all do it. When strength training, you have to retrain your brain to stop this. Holding your breath as you strength train, lift weights, or work out is dangerous. It can actually cause your blood pressure to spike rapidly and, in some cases, cause you to lose consciousness. Just breathe.
- **Rest:** You will notice sore and stiff muscles during strength training. This is normal, so we work on one muscle group, rest it, and move on to a different muscle group the following day. A good rule of thumb is to rest that muscle group for 24 to 48 hours before

returning to it. This will prevent injury as well

- **Use correct form:** Why should we use the proper form when training? First, if you use incorrect forms, you will hurt yourself. Second, if you don't use the correct form, you will be working out for no reason. That is right; you will see zero results. This is why it is always best and wise to begin your strength training by booking a few sessions with someone that is professionally trained. They will be able to show and teach you all the perfect forms you need to reach the goals you have set.

- **Listen to your body:** When lifting weights, it is normal to feel a bit stiff after a workout—it is a part of strength training. That being said, if you're hurt or injured, working out through the pain is never advisable. Stabbing or sharp pain indicates that you may have damaged a muscle or joint. If you feel discomfort or pain, you absolutely need to stop strength training. If the pain persists beyond two days or prohibits you from sleeping or doing typical daily tasks, seek medical attention.

I close my laptop with a new spark. The entire time I am getting ready for bed, I can picture it—me, Franny

Russo—bench pressing my way out of retirement!

A LOVE-HATE RELATIONSHIP WITH YOUR TRAINER!

I wake to what can only be described as a rooster being choked out by a dolphin underwater. When I hear it, I believe I am dreaming until I hear Robbie from the next room. "What the actual fried chicken is that noise?"

The next thing I hear, I will hold close to my heart forever—because I am that twisted.

"Franny, I have a problem, I have sprained me bloody snatch basket," Robbie said; in her Irish accent, she saves for times she is in pain.

I felt a pop, then burst out a sound that could only be described as a cackle. "Shit, there goes my snatch basket too, Robbie," I say, hoping to calm her.

I hear keys rattling in the front door, knowing Nora is about to burst through, glowing while eating her granola and ready for round two. "What are you two both still doing in bed, we are going to be late!" Nora yells before I have a chance, informing Nora we are out of commission, what with our sprained snatch baskets and all.

"Tribe, as much as I love all your colorful terminology for the vagina, I will roll you into that vehicle myself if need be, now grab your bathing suits and let's go," Nora states.

"Whoa, back it up Mary Poppins, what is it that just fell out your mouth?" Robbie is now on her feet.

Apparently, Marco has sent us all a text bright and early, already anticipating our sore muscle situation, and is ordering our session to be in the pool today. "Someone, please text him. We are going to be over 30 minutes late. My razor and I are going to need a moment," Robbie shuffles off to the shower.

Once we all arrive at the gym, we get our suits on, ready to hit the water, then Marco asks for an assessment of our pain as we get into the pool. He is specific about how we are truly feeling. He runs down some specific questions regarding what we all chose to eat for dinner and breakfast today, ensuring we are hitting that fiber and water target. We are told there are different types of pain to look for, all general muscle fatigue and intense or sharp pain in one spot.

Marco educates us on how to spot an injury, and that is what would cause severe pain in one muscle or joint. "In these instances, you should always stop all forms of exercise and strength training until you have it looked at by medical professionals," Marco tells us.

"When you feel pain and stiffness all over your body after a workout, this is something else entirely. So, what is causing that post-exercise pain is called delayed onset muscle soreness, or DOMS for short" (Tucker & Sgobba, 2021).

Marco continues to explain that DOMS occurs because small tears to our muscle fibers arise while we strength train or work out. It is those tiny microtears that cause all the pain and inflammation. He further explains that usually, the pain starts 12 to 24 hours post-workout and subsides around 48 to 72 hours afterward (Tucker & Sgobba, 2021).

"Holy crap on a cracker Marco, are you telling me that every time we come to one of your sessions, we are going to be tearing up our muscles?" Robbie spouts.

Marco assures us that this process is how we build muscle. "You see, when your muscle fibers start to build back up after these tears, they come back even stronger. It truly is normal and a part of the strength-building and new muscle growth process," Marco passionately states.

"So I feel we are back to the no pain no gain mantra all over again," I say.

"No, actually because more muscle pain, or DOMS, does not equate to faster or better muscle growth (Marturana Winderl & Braithwaite, 2020)," he assures me. "If you think about it, if you push yourself and are sore, you won't want to work out and will skip sessions," Marco continues. He explains that slow and steady always wins. Nobody is motivated or committed to strength training if they are in constant pain.

"I brought you all to the water today for a reason," Marco confesses. "It can be so easy to wake up sore and convince yourself to stay in bed, but this is a mistake," Marco says, looking us all in the eye.

He continues to tell us all that when our muscles are sore, they need us to move. The thought process is to wrap them up all cozy and let them rest, but that will cause them to seize and take even longer to heal. Moving them, even a little, will get the oxygen moving to that sore muscle and allow it to heal faster. Marco states that getting us in the water takes the weight off our joints, having us feel "weightless" but allowing us to still move our bodies.

Marco continues to tell us that strength training in the pool offers excellent benefits because the pool water is heavier than air. "The water is offering resistance against you, acting as your weight," Marco explains.

We are fully engaged as he continues, telling us how the added resistance of the water burns calories fast, uses all the muscles, and the buoyancy of the water supports our joints (Cronkleton, 2019).

Marco hands us foam dumbbells, used explicitly for water strength training as we continue to be educated. The foam in these dumbbells is buoyant and causes resistance when trying to keep them underwater. Marco now has us in the water at shoulder height with our arms at our sides and our elbows tight to our sides. Our palms are facing up and curling those foam weights while in the water. "Nice and slow, ladies, and just continue five reps per side as we chat," Marco instructs.

Marco continues to tell us that it is essential to remember the weights you use on land work your muscles against gravity as you raise them, but in the water, the resistance is the opposite. The dumbbells Marco has us use in the pool are designed to withstand our efforts when we lower them. He continues to explain that the larger the foam floats on our aquatic dumbbells, the more resistance we will experience.

"Ladies, your next, most important step is hydration, I have you swimming in the water, but I am going to need you drinking it like it is going to save the world," Marco says firmly.

Marco tells us of some research that shows a connection between dehydration, muscle soreness, and DOMS. It simply stated that if dehydration can increase soreness, then hydration can minimize it (Marturana Winderl & Braithwaite, 2020).

The study's leading theory is that water assists in flushing out the majority of the waste products. When our muscles break down, it is then that they release these waste products and toxins. If they are not filtered out of our body, they cause soreness in our muscles (Marturana Winderl & Braithwaite, 2020). So drink that water, filter out those toxins and waste, so all's right with your body.

As we continue our workout in the pool, I begin to notice my muscles relaxing. After a mere 15 minutes, I can move without pain, and my range of motion is back to normal. With my osteoporosis the way it is, mornings are difficult for me. A typical day would find me struggling until midday to accomplish basic tasks such as opening jars, tying my own shoes, and typing client notes. Yet today, after this time in the water, I already feel loose and am experiencing less pain.

"Before wrapping up today ladies, I want to give you one last key tip," Marco remarks.

Marco is passionate about the entire body and how what we feed it will also impact our muscles.

"Protein is an important nutrient for not only building, but also maintaining our muscles." Marco starts, "What most don't know is that protein is also important in the recovery of your muscles after you workout," He states with a kid's passion on Christmas morning.

He continues to inform us that we should always eat the required amount of protein to prevent soreness after our workouts. Those who work out should aim for roughly 1.4 to 2 grams of protein for every kilogram of body weight.

"To break that down, let's use Nora as an example," Marco suggests. "She is an active person who weighs approximately 155 pounds, so she should aim for 95 to 136 grams of protein per day, split across all her meals," Marco explains.

"If you reviewed your homework last night you would have found a few recipes to try, and because we are focusing on muscles and recovery, I was heavy on protein."

- tofu
- lean meats and poultry
- beans, peas, and lentils

- pork and wild game
- fish and shellfish
- peanuts and almonds
- nuts and seeds
- lower fat dairy products
- lean cuts of beef
- fortified soy beverages
- eggs

Marco rounded out our water-logged workout by reiterating the importance of sleep. "I cannot stress enough the need for rest and proper sleep to allow your muscles to rest and heal."

As we dragged our bodies from the water, we all admitted we felt refreshed and not as sore as when we started our day. On our way past Marco's office, Robbie popped her head inside, determined to leave him with a thought for the day. "Marco, you need to add an important note to the benefits of working out in the water," she begins.

"Oh, what is that Miss. Robbie?" as he has taken to affectionately calling her.

"You can fart all you want and nobody even notices!"

We all leave Marco with that bombshell of knowledge as we head off, considering day two a huge victory!

6

IS THIS HELL?

We have traveled through the Sahara desert, climbed Mt. Fuji, and traversed the Great Wall of China—I am startled awake by a dream or a nightmare; I am not sure which yet. The tribe decided that after reaching six months of strength training, we should enter *The Amazing Race—Over 50 Edition*.

Let me catch you up. All of us have been hard at work on this strength training for exactly four weeks today. Every last one of us has had moments of misery, victory, defeat, and celebration. We have bitched, complained, laughed, moaned, and groaned through it all. I am still scratching my head, trying to figure out how we got this far. Today we all have appointments with our doctors since starting strength training, and Robbie has to head back to New York City. We have kept her long enough from her love, Julie, and her other commitments. It is a big day, so let's get started.

MY EYELASHES HURT!

"Day 30 Marco, and I am limping in here like I am 101!" Robbie began. "I shit you not, my arm was shaking so bad trying to put on mascara this morning—were you aware eyelashes could hurt?"

She barely finished her sentence when Marco spits his coffee clear across the room. "You would think I'd be used to this tribe by now, wouldn't you?"

Like he always does when he is about to tell us something serious, Marco folds his arms across his expansive chest. He then asks us to all take a seat, which I am always happy to do at the gym. He continued explaining that he did not promise to "whip us into shape" within a set time frame.

"If you meet a trainer or a product that makes those promises, you should walk away," He continues.

He informs us that no one-size-fits-all program can determine how long it needs to get you in shape because every human body is different. Because of this, no trainer can look you in the eye and tell you that magical number. He continues telling us all that they should say this is now a lifestyle. It isn't a start-and-stop type of deal. If you want to live longer by being healthy, you must adapt strength training into your life —forever!

"That is all fine and good Marco, but is there a magic number for when I should be able to put on my mascara without shaking?" Robbie pipes up again.

"No, not a magic number," Marco answers, "30 days isn't much time for your body to understand this new change, but I would suggest easing up on the amount of arm weights you are using and see if that makes a difference. Remember, always listen to your body," he answers.

IT'S ARM DAY, AND I NEED TO LIFT MY WINE GLASS, MARCO!

Tonight we intend to celebrate. Thirty days of strength training may seem like peanuts to most, but this is a Herculean event for this tribe. Between the emotional roller-coaster moments and the fact that we must say goodbye to Robbie, we will be clinking glasses.

"Marco, it is arm day, and I will need to lift my wine glass tonight—more than once!" Nora says, looking him dead in the eye so she knows he understands.

"No worries Nora, it has been 72 hours since we last worked arms on you, which is the optimal recovery time for muscles" (Fitness 19, 2021).

Marco continues, explaining that giving your muscle groups 72 hours of rest will allow for muscle growth and recovery without risking injury from overtraining or under-recovery (Fitness 19, 2021).

He also wants to remind us that while we are allowing a set of muscle groups to recover on those down days, we shouldn't be ignoring them. Lactic acid builds up in dormant muscles, contributing to pain and stiffness. We still want to avoid overusing them, but we want to move them. So get out and go for a nice walk to use your legs and back muscles. Yoga is an excellent exercise to stretch muscles in the entire body and rid them of toxins and lactic acid (Fitness 19, 2021).

WHY IS MY ASS STILL BIG, MARCO?

Social media entered our world almost 30 years ago —I'll let you sit with that momentarily. One of its many negative impacts on every generation is the instant gratification bubble it has created. The "I want it now" mentality the internet has brought us is over the top. We no longer have to wait for much in life. Craving a cheeseburger at 2:00 a.m.? Uber Eats can have that at your doorstep in under 15 minutes. Dying for a new book to read? Amazon can deliver that to you that same day. Is it any wonder that we expect a gym or a trainer to work those same miracles?

"Marco, don't get me wrong, I enjoy my luscious booty, but I did think I'd be bouncing a quarter off it by now," Robbie inquires, very seriously.

"Have you tried?" I asked. We all burst out into laughter, but in all seriousness, she is waiting for an answer.

"Like most, you want tangible answers and numbers, I understand," Marco answers.

Marco decides to take a scientific approach to ensure we understand everything behind building muscle. He breaks it down the following way.

When our body builds muscle, it repairs those micro-traumas in our muscle fibers. Those DOMS we spoke of earlier. Below is a breakdown of this complex process (Capritto, 2022):

1. Our muscles are made up of thousands of tiny muscle fibers.
2. When you lift weights or do any strength training, your muscles get slight injuries within those fibers.

3. As you rest your muscles, your body will start repairing those damaged muscle cells.

4. The repair process requires combining torn muscle fibers back together and laying down new proteins in each muscle cell.

5. Now, the repair process makes your muscles grow into bigger and stronger forms.

This process includes your nervous, circulatory, and endocrine systems, as they all contribute to muscle repair and growth (Capritto, 2022).

"So what I am hearing Marco, is that in all good time, I will be able to bounce that quarter off my booty. I just need to be patient." Robbie announces.

"Yes, Robbie, that is indeed what I am saying," Marco says, finishing up his speech.

DAMN! FRANNY RUSSO JUST BENCH PRESSED 60 POUNDS!

Hands down, the biggest obstacle our tribe faced during these four weeks was motivation. That first week was a breeze. We had our new workout gear, we had our new trainer, and we had the newness of it all. But when life gets in the way, as it usually does, our priorities begin to shift. If we were having dinner to celebrate a family member's birthday, we would stay out later than usual and curse at that morning workout alarm. But, by week three, if we were presented with a more appealing invitation, it was next to impossible to turn it down.

The only thing that kept us on track was my surgery. Of course, we are well aware of the severity of our health concerns, but with my upcoming surgery date looming, we all just yelled the word "surgery," and back to the gym we would go.

The question remains, how do we get and stay motivated to keep ourselves on this healthy, strength training journey?

"This is such a great question," Marco answers, eager to start.

"There is actually science behind it. There are five basic steps to making anything you want to do a habit. If you follow the five steps below, it will become an automatic habit in your life, much like brushing your teeth or putting on deodorant."

They are as follows (Milkman, 2021):

- **Set a solid goal:** When forming a habit, you must set a specific goal. For example, stating that you want to get in shape is too vague. Zero in on why you want to get in shape. If you phrase it like, "I want to strength train to heal faster from surgery," you are being specific.

- **Make a detailed plan:** This is an extension of the above, but your plan needs to be detailed to completion. Know where you are to begin, the steps in the middle, and how it ends. If this is a lifestyle change, be sure you know what needs to change to make it happen. No stone is left unturned.

- **It needs to be exciting to repeat:** We are always excited when we start something new. We tend to forget to factor in the middle when things get dull or difficult. We also look for the fastest way to achieve our goals. This sets us up for failure from the start. Do your research and find out how to get the desired results, not just the fastest way to get there. Now that you know it may take some time, get creative and incorporate some fun and exciting things to keep you interested. This could mean trying yoga or Zumba to mix it up when it comes to working out.

- **Be flexible:** To have a successful habit-building process, you must rely on frequent, repeating behaviors. However, if you become too rigid with time and don't allow any flexibility in your schedule, all it takes is one wrench in that schedule to throw it all off. Don't be afraid of mixing up those workout times a few times a week after that first month. This tricks your brain into believing you have the ability to be flexible if need be.

- **Tell everyone:** You may have heard that if you are trying to accomplish something, keep it to yourself. In this case, tell all your friends and family when establishing a new habit. We are influenced by those in our circle, and good habits are always contagious, so pay attention to who you surround yourself with. For example, if you want to begin strength training, it wouldn't be wise to start working out with a nephew or friend who has been weightlifting for 10 years. Keep it all relative.

Marco wraps up his educational bit on forming habits, and I can feel my anticipation building. Of course, the tribe doesn't know it yet, but Marco and I have a huge surprise for them.

"Marco, as a nurse, I appreciate the science behind all of this. My brain now understands much more of this," Nora remarks.

I stand up and start leaving the room, and I can hear the girls asking each other what I'm doing. "Oh, I believe it is time," Marco says, directing both Nora and Robbie to follow him. I feel my heartbeat quicken because I know they are right behind me with no idea what is happening.

Marco stands behind me as I sit on the bench press, ready to spot me. "Franny, for the love of all things orgasmic, *what* are you doing?" Robbie spews concern with each word coming out of her voice. Nora has come as close as she possibly can. "I hope one of you has your camera ready," Marco says.

What the tribe doesn't know is that ever since I saw that woman on the front page of the article Marco sent that first night, I wanted to be her. I wanted to feel the power that comes from bench pressing. I wanted to feel the power that comes from gaining muscle. So I spoke to Marco privately about my dream and goals. He has been working with me secretly to achieve this.

"Are you ready ladies?" I ask before blowing their freaking minds.

I wrap my gloved hands around that cold iron bar, and goosebumps climb up my forearms, straight up my spine. I immediately hear a voice in my head that I believe belongs to my badass Nana. *"You show em' Franny bear."*

With Marco spotting and my tribe watching me with eyes wide open, I successfully bench-pressed 60 pounds. Of course, I farted loudly, but it didn't matter because, at that moment, I was so damn proud of myself. Me, Franny freakin' Russo just benched 60 pounds, people! About to be 55 years young, and look at me, go!

As I sat up, my eyes landed on my tribe sisters, tears streaming down their faces as they rushed over to wrap their arms around me. "You smell like ass, but did you actually just do that?" Robbie says through a snotty nose and tear-stained face.

Nora, continuing to sob, finally finds her words. "Franny, I am almost speechless but I have never been more proud of you than I am at this moment."

Then it happened. Applause from every person in the gym. Millennials, gym rats, seniors, every person just stopped their day and celebrated with me. And with that, I am a sweaty, sobbing mess.

These are the moments we hold on to. The days we can barely get out of bed because of pain. The days we are facing scary surgery and recovery. The days we know aging will change our bodies and our minds. So hold on to your victories and use them to motivate you.

It has been a long and emotional day. After we wrapped up at the gym, we had a wonderful dinner at our favorite restaurant to celebrate the accomplishments of our tribe. We just kept saying how we couldn't believe we stuck to our plan and went to the gym daily for an entire month. After dinner, we had to take Robbie to the airport. Plenty of hugs and tears as we said our goodbyes as usual, but we know her next visit is planned soon.

Marco already helped Robbie find a fantastic trainer in her area to help keep her on track back at home. He plans to follow up with Robbie's trainer to ensure Robbie has no slip-ups in the next four weeks. While Nora and I will continue training with Marco for the next four weeks. After that time, we were confident to go at it alone. Of course, that was after a few conversations with Marco, where he agreed that we would have the tools and support to stick to our 20 to 30 minutes of strength training exercises daily.

Marco has recommended a great physiotherapist for me for post-surgery that I intend to use. After that, the plan is to continue and maintain what is working and start turning our attention to diet and gut health.

7

DOCTOR VISIT DAY

W hen this adventure began, every one of us had reservations. Nora was excited to get both Robbie and me into the gym and work out with her, but even she was hesitant about working on her mental health. I would be lying if I didn't tell you that I am stunned by how amazing I feel. I won't admit that to Nora yet; maybe I will write it on her birthday card. The first month we did this as a tribe, it wouldn't have worked any other way. But then, Robbie had to get back to New York, and it was Nora and me while Robbie adopted a new program back home.

We have been worried about how that transition would go. So we scheduled a Zoom meeting with her once a week, and now, four weeks later, she is flying back. Robbie's doctor is in Arizona, so she will be meeting with her tomorrow when Nora and I meet with our doctors.

"Franny, don't you think that sign is going just a little too far?" Nora asks me as I stand in the airport with it high above my head. It reads, and I quote, "Happy Prison Release Day!"

Robbie saw it and bent over in laughter, so I say—*win!*

AN APPLE A DAY?

We roll up to one of our favorite Mexican restaurants, and as always, my heart feels whole and my soul complete because the tribe is together. After we smother Robbie in hugs and love, we get down to business—ordering food!

I can tell you another thing about us women, we are creatures of habit. As much as Nora loves adventure, all three of us are not lovers of change. So, I was in shock as I saw us order food and drinks, hand over the menus, and not even notice.

"Hey tribe, did you see what we did out of habit just now?" I ask as they glance up from the salsa.

"What did you observe?" Nora asks inquisitively.

None of us ordered "the usual" jalapeno poppers, chicken strips, and loaded potato skins—all loaded with calories, high in carbs, and low in protein. I went on to explain that we never visit this restaurant without ordering drinks by the bottle or pitcher, and without hesitating, we each ordered a single glass. I look across the table, and Robbie's mouth is still hanging open. Nora is beaming with pride for all of us.

I am the only one bold enough to say it like it is. "I will be honest, I thought Marco was talking out his ass about this forming a habit shit," I confess. "Yet here we are doing things opposite of what we've been doing for more than 20 years without thinking about it or missing it," I continued.

Nora begins, "Tribe, you know I was open about how dark some of my days were leading up to this, so I need to thank you for doing this with me. Not even I knew how much I needed it," she went on. Nora explained how she fought Marco in the beginning because reducing the training she was doing made her feel weak and old, much like the rest of her life. However, she leaned into the process and trusted Marco, and now, she feels stronger because she isn't waking up sore and stiff, so she isn't skipping days. Her mental health is showing signs of improving too. Having the ability to see she can have control over this next chapter in her life has helped significantly.

Fear can prevent us from seeing what is behind doors in the next part of our life. If you are afraid, kick it open instead. Showing that fear has no place in your life, you may be shocked that what is behind the fear was what you were looking for. You can be in control and determine the levels of peace, quiet, calm, excitement, and thrill you want in life. If you are not excited about kicking the door down, gather your tribe, and if you don't have one, think about creating one because there is strength in numbers. If it is just you, then create your tribe of knowledge, wisdom, power, and strength. Always look back on the scary and intimidating things you have accomplished up until now. Draw on that energy now. You've got this.

"I came into this believing I would fail," Robbie confesses. "Then I would watch you two and be encouraged by both of you, if I would have packed my ass back onto that plane then I would have to explain to my partner why I failed at something again," she says, with the words stuck in her throat with emotion.

Robbie runs down the line of significant losses and failures she has endured, but she wants this to be her turning point. She wants her grown children to see she is committed to being around for a long time for her grandbabies. Robbie wants her partner to see she is committed to their life together. But, most importantly, she says, with passion streaming down her cheeks, she wants her own self to finally know she matters.

We wrap our arms around our tribe sister. We know she understands our love for her, but we love knowing she gets it. We love knowing she broke through some old messed-up trauma and came out this side, all from strength training with her tribe.

"I know you all did this for me because I was terrified." I confide in my tribe that this strength training gig was intended to get me in shape for surgery. My tribe sisters are these types of friends. I explained that I would never quit, no matter how hard, because they did this for me. As I feel that familiar lump in my throat, I lean down and take a sip of water. We ask someone at the next table to take a picture of us so we always remember this night.

We all climb into bed nice and early—doctor visits bright and early.

HEY DOC, IT'S ME, FRANNY

What's up with the paper gowns in the doctor's office? Why? When I am anxious, I sweat! Do you know what happens to paper when it gets wet? You guessed it, it disintegrates before your eyes. I am convinced I will sit here with confetti covering my nipples before this doctor walks in.

I am so anxious. *Why am I so nervous? Stop worrying so much, Franny. You have been doing all the right things since your last visit! I mutter to myself.*

The door handle rattles, and I sit up straight in my moist, paper gown. The doctor flashes me his ultra-white toothy grin. "Good morning Ms. Russo. How are you today?" He asks, reaching for my hand. I apologize for the damp palm and the half-missing attire and respond that I am fine, which is the obligatory response in these situations.

I had been sent for blood labs and imaging on my hips prior to this appointment, so we would have a current understanding of what was happening within this temple, what others call a body. The doctor looks at me from behind the screen with the biggest smile. "Your strength trainer has been in touch with me, and Franny, I must say…."

I rudely interrupt him by blurting out. "Did he tell you, gosh I wanted to tell you… I bench pressed 60 pounds and doctor, it was amazing!"

"That is impressive and you should be proud, but no he didn't tell me," the doctor said.

I decided to let the man speak as he continued to inform me that my blood panel told the true story of the last eight weeks of my hard work. For example, my blood sugar on my previous blood panel was 16, and today is nine—within the normal range. As well, my cholesterol has dropped. He went into detail on this one for a bit.

My doctor was concerned about my cholesterol levels, which affect our heart health. He and Marco had been chatting about ways to get this number to drop. I had no idea that strength training could play a role in this at all. Because my hip is causing some mobility issues, cardio isn't ideal for me at this time, and cardio can lower cholesterol fast. My doctor told me of a study done in 2019 where people who lifted weights one hour each week but, like me, couldn't do any cardio. They had a 65% less risk for heart attack or stroke than someone who didn't lift (Comprehensive Spine Institute, 2021).

"Doc, are you telling me that my cholesterol has dropped, too?" I finally asked.

"Franny, I am so happy to report that your cholesterol numbers are now in the range that makes my heart happy," He says, smiling.

We wrap up our session with a surgery date. As scary as this all seems, I now know my surgery will be quick, and I am not afraid of recovery any longer. I know I have built up the muscles I need to support my mobility and my recovery. My doctor informs me that his timeline originally had me on track for a three-month recovery, and now, four weeks later, he feels I will be well on my way in less than 2 months.

We look at our calendars, and he is aware of the infamous tribe sister's birthday extravaganza trip we are booking. So he graciously agrees to schedule my surgery for two weeks after we return.

HELLO DOCTOR, NORA HERE

As Nora sits in the exam room of her doctor, she is still adjusting to the new office. Nora has recently changed her doctor down to Arizona full-time. As I mentioned, not one of us likes change, and Nora had her previous doctor for 15 years. It is common knowledge that nurses make terrible patients, and Nora herself will agree. Nurses visit a doctor when they've pretty much decided they can't treat the condition themselves.

Why do doctor's offices have to smell so ugh, Nora thinks to herself. She is tempted to spritz some of her body spray into the air to calm her nerves, knowing full well this is a "scent-free" environment. But the doctor walks in before her nerves get the best of her.

"It is so nice to see you again, Nora," the doctor reaches for Nora's hand to greet her. Now seated at the computer screen, the clicking of the keys and her information appear before his eyes. "Oh, this is fantastic. Definitely improvements from the last blood draw," he remarks.

"I didn't realize there were any issues; nothing was mentioned to me," Nora says with a raised eyebrow.

The doctor continues, stating that certain things begin to appear as we age, and unless the numbers are high, we won't mention them. "They were just beginning to creep up there, but now, they are all the way back at the bottom: glucose, cholesterol, you name it! So I am pleased with how your blood work is looking, but tell me how you are feeling, I know last time we met, you mentioned stiff and sore muscles, as well as fatigue."

Nora lowered her head slightly, took a breath to center herself, and let it all out. Then, she confided in her new doctor, telling him about the life transition she currently finds herself in. By the time she is done, she is shocked to see that 30 minutes have passed, and not once did the doctor interrupt her. "I am so sorry. I have eaten up so much of your time," she apologizes as she stands.

"You need to stop apologizing so much," the doctor answers back. "It is my job to listen and help, and that is what I do."

Nora's doctor takes action and starts by congratulating her on taking the first step by talking to him. They agree that Nora is now on a great path with her new therapist and her strength training path. However, her bloodwork shows some markers of the stress she is holding. She is experiencing anxiety and feels this is her next hurdle to overcome.

While they work together with her therapist, he recommends a referral to a nutritionist to see if something is going on with her gut health. Women ignore symptoms within their bodies that can cause anxiety, stress, hair loss, insomnia, and about 50 other symptoms that can all come from what we put in our bodies. Nora's doctor knows she still has work to do and that it takes time. Nobody wants to leave an appointment knowing their stressful symptoms will still linger for months or years. He further recommends she begins massage therapy once a week to reduce stress and anxiety. He also insists she finds a hobby she loves that is only for her. He wants her to allot one hour a week to that. Close out the world and give that to herself. He is there, and it is her decision to reach out if she would like medical intervention in the form of medication for anxiety at any time. Her doctor reminds her that stress is felt in the body, not just in the mind. "Your sore muscles are also caused by stress Nora, so during those more stressful times, it is okay to be gentle with yourself. Move those muscles, love yourself, and ask for all the help you deserve," he reaches out to shake her hand.

Nora continues to smile as she gathers herself from that very emotional appointment. Then finally, she will take it all in and heed the advice. "I like him. He knows his stuff," Nora mutters to herself as she exits the building.

ROBBIE, THE DOCTOR WILL SEE YOU NOW

Robbie is fiercely pacing—in that medical paper dress and *Ugg* boots. As the swooshing continues, she can feel the sweat run down the small of her back, and her first thought is, *Does this doctor need to be anywhere near my butt?* Robbie recalls the last time she was here because she felt attacked. Words flash across her visual field. Fat. Lazy. Diabetic. Unlike her two tribe sisters, she has secretly been convinced nothing she has done has made one ounce of difference to her health.

Just then, the doctor enters, and before he can even look up from his notes and greet her, she blurts out... "Doc, I am sweating like a wine bottle in the Sahara desert, so I will need you to just cut to the chase. I have been busting this fine ass of mine for the past two months, and I need you to validate if my hard work has paid off," Robbie continues, sweat now beading on her upper lip.

"Robbie, whatever you are doing, it is working. Now have a seat because your pacing makes me anxious," Robbie's doctor states. "Let's begin with your blood glucose number. When you visited me eight weeks ago, it was dangerously high at 21, and I am happy to report that today it is 11."

"Is this good, Doc?" Robbie asks.

The doctor explains to Robbie that she is no longer at risk of developing diabetes. The doctor further explains that he and her trainer have worked closely together because some types of strength training can cause spikes in your sugar if not careful. This tends to happen if you already have diabetes and do more aerobic workouts with heavy deadlifting. Marco kept her health issues in mind, so her strength training was not aerobic, and her repetitions were always under 12, thus preventing any spikes in her blood sugar (Oerum, 2020).

"One last thing, Robbie, I notice here on my screen that you haven't renewed your pain medication." The doctor points to her chart. Robbie's jaw hangs open as she reaches into her purse for what she has referred to as her lifeline in the past. Her pain medication is what keeps her in the game. The flare-ups she experiences from her osteoarthritis have kept her in bed for days before. She has been making excuses to avoid family vacations for fear of the swollen knees and limping they would notice. Yet today, she holds up a bottle still three-quarters full.

"Well smack my arse and call me Sally. This is a first, eh doc?" Robbie spouts as only Robbie does. Her tears welled up, which was completely unexpected.

The doctor places a hand on her shoulder and reminds her of her outstanding accomplishments. "You have worked through the pain, congratulations. You just proved the theory that most find more relief through movement than with medication—keep up this amazing work!"

Those with osteoarthritis need to remember one of the worst things we can do for our sore and stiff muscles is to keep them still. The lactic acid will build up and cause more pain. Any slow or small movement will help ease that pain (Comprehensive Spine Institute, 2021).

IT IS WINE O'CLOCK SOMEWHERE

It has been another long and emotional day for the tribe, and by the time they all gather for dinner, they are bursting at the seams to hear about all the doctor visits. They are all anticipating and hoping for the best without knowing how their individual appointments went. I mean, how can you celebrate excellent news if one of your tribe sisters was given crap news?

I am the first to arrive, a quality I pride myself on— always needing to be early. I also like being able to pick the best seat at the table and order appetizers for the table. Robbie had a few quick errands to wrap up before dinner, as she would be flying home in the morning. I quickly glance up to see Nora and, right behind her, Robbie, just as they enter the restaurant.

It takes one glance from all of us, and we squeal, hug, and sob in one big heap in the booth I knew would be perfect for this occasion. "Okay, wait, I have ordered a pitcher of skinny margaritas for the table, but I say let's cheer with this ice water because I can't wait to hear all this good news," I say, glass in the air.

We spent the next six hours reviewing all the fantastic stories from our healthcare team from today. We clink glasses over a dozen times, take multiple photos, and even call Marco on speakerphone to share our happiness.

We have two new dates to focus on, planning our celebratory birthday extravaganza and my upcoming surgery. I now look at both those dates with excitement. The following day, we do our usual sad goodbye at the airport as Robbie returns to her partner Julie in New York City. We will visit her next as we plan our huge birthday trip.

Tomorrow, we meet with Marco to discuss future plans, including post-surgery strengthening workouts and how we can use strength training to drop some of these pesky pounds.

8

IT IS TIME TO RE-EVALUATE

W hat a weekend! My heart is whole, knowing that not only myself but my tribe is healthy and on the right track. Today, Nora and I are meeting with Marco to discuss these next four weeks.

MODIFIED EXERCISES FOR SURGERY RECOVERY

What a weekend! My heart is whole, knowing that not only myself but my tribe is healthy and on the right track. Today, Nora and I are meeting with Marco to discuss these next four weeks.

Returning to the gym is so odd because I never thought I would open these doors, making it feel comfortable and familiar. "Hello, tribe," Marco greets us at the entrance of his office. We usher ourselves in and have a seat. "Nora, you are more than welcome to get started on your workout if you wish. I will cover a few things with Franny this morning before she starts," Marco states.

Nora jumps up excitedly and heads off to her happy place as I settle in to take notes.

Marco gets started with a breakdown of specific exercises designed for me to begin the day after my surgery. He notices the raised eyebrows and wrinkled forehead. "I know this sounds intense Franny, but the sooner we get you moving, the sooner we get blood and oxygen flowing to the joint and you will feel less pain and back to your normal self," Marco pipes up.

I nod so he knows I understand. "Tell me what I need to do, and I will get it done."

The list Marco gives me is as follows (Winternitz, 2016):

Glute Squeezes: Your gluteus maximus muscles are located at the back of your hip and help support and control your hip joints. When doing this exercise, you should:

1. Lay flat on your back and extend your legs.

2. Next, gently squeeze your butt for five seconds, then release it.

Glute squeezes aim to strengthen your gluteus muscles without worrying about putting any stress on your new joint. Try 10 repetitions and then rest.

Thigh Squeezes: Your quadriceps muscles are located on the front of your thigh, and their job is to support and control your hip joints. To perform this exercise, you should:

- Lie flat on your back, legs extended.
- Squeeze your quadriceps muscles—located on the front of your thigh.
- While squeezing, your leg should be straight.
- Hold for five seconds.

The purpose of this exercise will be the strengthening of the quadriceps muscles without causing unnecessary movement or putting any strain on your hips.

Ankle Pumps: We want to ensure we also move and exercise the muscles in our lower legs. This helps maintain our strength and improves blood circulation, both essential for healing.

1. Once again, lie on your back with your legs extended and your ankle raised slightly on a towel or blanket.
2. Flex your foot, pushing your heel away from your body, and point your toe up and toward your body.
3. Hold this position for five seconds.
4. Now, while pointing your toe, move your heel toward the calf and your toes pointing away from the body.
5. Hold this position for five seconds.

The reason for this exercise is to stimulate blood flow within your leg and strengthen your lower leg. This combined will help support your new hip.

Hip Abductions: Any abduction exercises require moving your limb away from your body. This reclined hip abduction requires you to:

1. Lie on your back with your legs extended.
2. Keep your surgical leg straight, and your toes pointed up. Then slide your leg to the side, slowly moving away from the center of your body.
3. Move your surgical leg back to the center. Don't move it past the center because you don't want to risk dislocation.

4. Always be sure to keep the other leg extended and perfectly straight.

These hip abduction exercises can be done standing up once you feel strong. When ready, your physical therapist can also show you how to add resistance using strength resistance bands.

These hip abduction exercises will help stabilize your pelvis and strengthen your new joint.

"Wait, Marco! These are the same exercises you started with me on the first day of strength training."

Marco replies with a smile, "That is correct Franny, having strengthened those muscles pre-surgery will put you way ahead of schedule with recovery and make the exercises easier after surgery."

"I feel much better knowing these exercises and what I'm doing the second I come out of surgery. Thank you Marco for going above and beyond, as usual. I feel confident and fully prepared too!"

STRENGTHENING EXERCISES TO ASSIST IN WEIGHT LOSS

The tribe's next goal is shedding some of the extra pounds we have been carrying. When we first met with

Marco, he asked us to create a list of wants for our health journey and prioritize them. Weight loss was number one for myself and Robbie. Marco quickly made us understand that by doing what was necessary to bring our glucose levels and cholesterol levels down, our weight would follow. Most times, people get so caught up in the number on the scale that all the other important health issues take a back burner. Now that we have our pressing health issues in check, we are getting educated on why, at our age, this weight issue is such a damn headache!

Nora has helped explain why, as we age, our metabolism slows down. Once women hit those fabulous 50s, they lose muscle, which causes their metabolism to slow (Cramer, 2018).

"Okay, but why is it that men escape this affliction so well?" Robbie asks, demanding answers. We have had her join us in this meeting via Zoom, so she doesn't miss any pertinent information.

"Great question," Marco speaks up. He continues to explain that men do not escape this one. It is menopause that causes us to experience it at an accelerated rate. "You can thank the lack of estrogen, ladies. This targets fat directly to your midsection, unlike men," Marco explains (Cramer, 2018). He tells us the more significant issue is that added fat leads to severe problems like type 2 diabetes, heart attack, and stroke (Cramer, 2018).

"Well isn't this just tickety-boo." I hear Robbie from across the country.

Marco continues, telling us we are all on the right path, reminding us how far we have come since meeting him. "I meet all types of people, and most ignore all my suggestions, instead joining all the latest fad diets." He strongly encourages us to continue doing what we are in strength training.

Our trainer is passionate about educating us. He wants us to know that cardio used to be what we all were taught to burn fat. Now, they know strength training does a fantastic job of this. The question is how? It increases your muscle mass, which burns more calories when you are at rest, which now we know increases your metabolism (Cramer, 2018).

Knowing us the way he does, Marco anticipates we will want a few new strength training exercises targeted at weight loss. "Tribe, I have put together five specific strength training exercises that are aimed at dropping pounds," Marco states. He informs us that some use specific weights, and some use our body weight as resistance. He instructs us to start incorporating the following into our regular program at our own comfort level (Higuera, 2019).

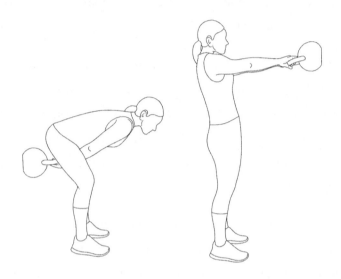

Kettlebell Swings

Be prepared for a complete and challenging full-body workout. This exercise is designed to increase your heart rate while building arm and leg strength. After adopting this exercise into your routine, you should see a more muscular core.

1. 1Using a two-handled kettlebell, do a full swing with both hands for a full 20 seconds.
2. Rest your body for a total of eight seconds.
3. Aim for 8 to 10 repetitions.

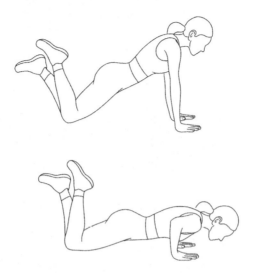

Pushups

These are a great way to stabilize your core, build excellent upper body strength, and increase muscle mass in those arms.

When beginning, start with just three sets of 10 reps. After completion, rest for one minute between each set. You can then increase your reps as you feel your strength improving.

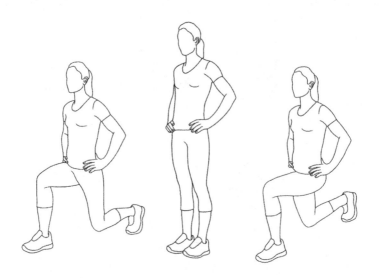

Lunges

Lunges provide plenty of options and flexibility because they can be done with weights or without, and forward or backward. You can add weights by holding a kettlebell or a weight plate close to your chest.

You should aim for a complete set of 8 to 12 lunges per leg. Do one leg, then rest as needed.

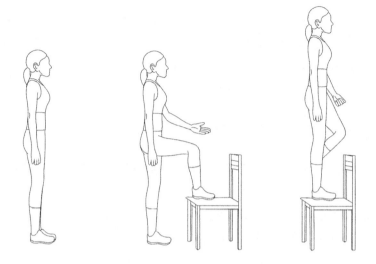

Step-ups

These are perfect for strengthening your legs and stabilizing your core and lower back muscles. Start with a small step height—no more than six to nine inches—then move up to a higher elevation—12 to 18 inches as you feel confident.

• Do five sets of five, completing 10 reps on each side.

When ready to make it a bit more challenging, you can add extra weight by holding a kettlebell or weight plate close to your chest. This will increase your heart rate, burning those calories fast.

I must admit, this new information from Marco has me excited about working out again. I am shocked to even think about these things. Me, Franny Russo, a gym rat! I love how I am feeling and, dare I say... looking.

WHAT YOU NEED TO KNOW AS YOU AGE

It's nighttime, and my phone rings while I am curled up on the couch. It was Nora, and we had a great chat about this entire adventure. Our most significant focus is how much we have learned about our bodies.

"You would think, being a nurse, I would have had more knowledge about this aging business." Nora says with a slight chuckle.

"I believe, as always, you are so caught up in making sure everyone else is good you ignore what is changing in your own temple," I quickly answer, knowing she gets it.

We spent almost three hours really digging deep. We realize how much a woman's body endures, from puberty to menopause. So why do we go through all of this and seldom discuss it? It is terrifying, exhausting, and annoying, yet we feel the need to go it alone. Every one of these transitions causes severe issues with our health. First, our hormones skyrocket, then they take a dive and then vacate our bodies. As women in our fifties and older, we need to have a more open dialogue about these issues to take better care of our health.

Before starting this adventure, I had no clue that I could strength train to lower my blood sugar and cholesterol, drop weight, and feel like a badass. Yet, here I am!

9

CELEBRATE EVERY VICTORY

One thing has held true throughout all of this. We celebrated everything. The first time Robbie did a squat without farting, I busted out actual pom poms right there in the gym. The first time I managed to deadlift and not piss my pants, the girls finally took the adult diapers out of my trunk. I put them back in—better safe than sorry, I say. When Nora realized she was sleeping more than five hours a night and her stress was more manageable, Robbie and I wrote her a rap song. It was epic, and we now perform it for her countless times a week.

Marco was not left out of our celebration madness. We brought him a gift the week we realized we were down five pounds each. A t-shirt with all three of our gorgeous faces, and on the back, it stated, "honorary tribe member." I saw him wipe away several tears.

If you are anything like our tribe and know your strength training journey is going to start out miserable, you need to get ready to celebrate everything. If you don't, you are more likely to quit. It is okay if you are going this alone. I suggest setting the smallest goals and assigning prizes when you hit them. Do you love expensive specialty coffee? If you make it to the gym three days in a row, buy yourself one. Are you like me and love watching marathons on Netflix? If you blow off a fun event for a workout, reward yourself with two solid hours of your favorite show.

Just knowing you have a reward waiting for you is often enough incentive. The key is rewarding the small accomplishment along the way, not just the significant victories.

IT IS TIME TO PLAN THE "GREECE" CELEBRATION

"Celebrate good times; come on!" We cannot be friends if you are not singing the lyrics in your head right now. It is time, people—to celebrate the tribe in style! Soon it will be our 55th birthday, and plans are underway! Nora and I are just about to land in N.Y.C. as we figured it is only fair for us to visit Robbie this time as we hash out all the details and book this trip. Not to mention, what could be better than a trip to the Big Apple and exploring the sights and the glorious food?

Our flight landed on time, and I could not wait to wrap my arms around Robbie and Julie. Nora has been anxious the entire flight because she has been convinced since age 12 that she will perish in an airplane explosion. We grab our bags, and then I see it. The sign held high above Robbie's head reads, "*Welcome Home, Franny, I Picked Up Your Vagisil.*" I am on the floor laughing. Nora is 10 feet back, mortified, and the prize for best sign goes to Robbie!

We started planning our celebration trip to Greece at Robbie and Julie's chic New York apartment. We soon realized the last time we were planning a trip, the final decision came down to where we could lounge by a pool and do the least amount of walking. This trip would be different. Our dream destination has always been Greece, but we have always shot it down because of the walking we would have to do. Now, in the best shape of our lives since high school, we will be heading to Greece!

All three of us stop dead in our tracks as we hear ourselves mentioning that we won't have to feel guilty for missing gym time, as those hikes in the mountains will be great workouts. Robbie pipes up, "Listen to us, and who the heck are we?"

I quickly respond, letting the ladies know I have researched this topic as I remind Robbie that I have my surgery two weeks after we return.

I let them know I had a whole workout planned for all of us. I pulled it up on my laptop, showing them how we can use our full backpacks as kettlebells, pool noodles in the water for dumbbells, and yoga on the beach (Kamb, 2022). "I have us covered, ladies!" To say we are excited about this trip is an understatement.

With our trip planned to start in 3 weeks, Nora and I returned to Arizona to get packed and ready for our big trip to Greece. The 21 days passed quickly, and soon we would be packing for our 2-week trip. Nora and I will return to New York City to join Robbie at her place to catch the flight to Greece from John F. Kennedy Airport in New York City two days later. We are excited beyond belief to explore Greece with our new, energized, soon-to-be 55-year-old bodies!

HAPPY BIRTHDAY TO US AND HELLO
GREECE!

After the first glorious week with the turquoise waters, we noticed that we couldn't get enough of booking excursions, hikes, and tours. No more choosing to sit around, eat, and drink all day and night. Yes, there will be plenty of that, but we are also excited to explore the beautiful country.

As the night winds down, the tribe reflects on their previous diet and exercise failures and why this one was a success.

Robbie starts first. "Okay, I tried in the eleventh grade —the cabbage soup diet. For seven straight days, you eat nothing, absolutely nothing but cabbage soup," Robbie says with her nose curled up. "I could throw up just thinking about cabbage now." She continues to tell us about how she cannot eat cabbage to this day because of that diet trend.

I asked if it worked and if she had lost any weight. "What I lost was my dignity. Do you know what cabbage makes you do?" She asks before telling us how she farted so loud in the middle of science class. "Don't you all remember for the rest of that year, those kids called me 'bombs away' when I walked by?" Robbie recalled. She says, "I couldn't stop farting for a week and felt bloated the whole time, but I did lose 11 pounds."

Up next, Nora stated she was tasked with cooking for her entire family from a very young age. This created a love-hate relationship with food for Nora. She was too tired to eat when she cooked and cleaned for everyone else. This led her to find Slimfast, that super convenient meal you could drink. "My thought process was, if I can drink what I need quickly, I will have more time for my studies and chores. That lasted all of six months before I noticed my hair falling out, and then I fainted twice at school. My doctor said my blood work was a disaster because these drinks don't contain enough calcium and other nutrients children need", Nora informed us (Nunez, 2019).

"I did buy myself the *Thigh Master* after witnessing Suzanne Somers in her unitard flawlessly demon-strating how easily I could sculpt my thighs just like her," Nora commented. "I saved up for two months to purchase mine for $19.95, and let me tell you that no tenth-grade female with spaghetti arms and chicken legs could work that thing," Nora laughed. We all laughed hysterically at the thought of this. She was not wrong. I almost sheared off a nipple once trying to use one.

Okay, my turn. Do you all remember those machines that you would wrap a wide band around your butt and turn it on, and it would shake you like shake and bake chicken? It belonged to my grandmother. She called it her "slimming machine," although I don't know what it was called. Well, I had watched a movie as a young girl, and each morning, a well-dressed, stylish woman would start her day on this machine, and something stuck in my brain. From eighth to tenth grade, this is how my day ended. That is until Mark Alden saw me. He was hanging out with my brother and was using the facilities when he opened the wrong door. How does one even explain what he saw? I decided to go with "I had a medical condition," but I don't think he bought it. Regardless, I tossed the machine into the hallows of the basement, never to be used again.

Aside from that machine, please, I have done all the fad diets. Atkins, South Beach, NutriSystem, Weight Watchers, you name it, I've tried it. If you are now asking me why they didn't work, and this has, I believe it comes down to marketing. Everything we have tried previously was trying to sell us a product. This time, we invested in ourselves. So, to all of the readers out there who are on the fence about what to try next, if the "thing" you are considering insists you need one of their products to help you succeed, move along.

"Omgosh, that reminds me of the last two fad diets I tried. I would say three years ago I tried the baby food diet. It is exactly what it sounds like. You replace all your meals with jars of baby food in an attempt to control your portions. On day seven, I fainted at work;

three times. Mortified, I recall waking up surrounded by paramedics asking me my name. It was at the hospital I was told baby food does not have the nutrients and calories a full-grown adult needs," Robbie recalls.

"Did I learn my lesson? Hell no, because one year later I was all about the grapefruit diet. This involved me eating half a grapefruit with each meal and those meals are drastically reduced in portion size. I should start out by stating how much I despise citrus fruits, and most of all grapefruit. I stuck with it for 11 days and found myself dizzy, exhausted, and in need of more nutrients. That was it for me. I realized I was doing harm to my body by putting it through these fad diets. If I am meant to be fluffy, so be it. I do want to be healthy though," Robbie finishes.

During one of our famous wicnics (wine picnics), the ladies and I had an epiphany.

"I just realized something. While researching the topic of strength training, I uncovered enough information to put together a book. I want to thank both of you for encouraging me to follow through on this. Not to toot my own horn, but I believe I will be able to write a fantastic self-help book using our journey to strength training and I now will have a mission during my recovery," I stated with confidence.

STRENGTH TRAINING FOR WOMEN OVER 50 | 165

"Either this wine is making me feel inspired or you are Franny, but hear me out. After visiting my doctor and finding out how some of my health issues could be tied to my gut, I want to write a book on digestion and gut health," Nora states.

"That is a great idea. I mean, who do you think will hit #1 Best Seller first? Joking, it will be me obviously," I laughed.

"Well, I don't want to be left out of this publishing extravaganza, so I want to commit to writing a book as well. No clue what I will write about yet, but it is guaranteed to be a competition for Ms Franny's book!" Robbie says, slapping her knee.

"Robbie, I love this idea. There are so many topics you could write about. You love to talk about travel, cooking, and self-love. I have no doubt whatever you choose to write about will be amazing," Nora says.

"I am one proud friend at this moment. I love the idea of your books, Nora and Robbie. I believe you will find the perfect topics! I know we all thrive with friendly competition. I can see us now doing book tours and signings. Just don't forget who your real friends are when we are *Oprah* famous.

"Let's raise a glass, ladies, shall we?" Nora says as we watch the sun setting in the Mediterranean Sea.

"Cheers to us being 55 years young and in the best shape of our lives."

We all clink glasses, taking in the beautiful scenery that Greece has to offer us. The warm sea air kisses our cheeks, and the calm is felt all the way into our souls. This vacation is a celebration of our lives together. It is the pinnacle of our journey through life and the beginning of our next chapter.

As I look out over the brilliant white rooftops against the turquoise-blue water, my senses are stimulated, and I feel so alive. All this feels like a second chance at life, to live it on our terms. As we age, society starts telling us how to live. They think we should slow down, not take risks, wear sensible shoes, get to bed early, and behave. Who put them in charge of my temple? Remember what I said earlier, your ability, not your age, determines your decisions.

Soon we'll be headed back home, and this celebration will be one great memory that will last a lifetime and is well worth the work we put in to earn it. My next project will be to talk Robbie and Julie into moving to Arizona.

CONCLUSION

Throughout this book, you have watched all three of us fail. From the beginning, you watched Robbie almost throat-punch her doctor when she was convinced he called her a fat cow. She was sure this would be a waste of her time from the start. Slowly but with intention, she went from farting during her workouts to needing next to no pain medication. Robbie now realizes it was worth the effort.

We witnessed our superhero, Nora, and her mental health in the toilet, to be honest. She finally noted that her stress was a big reason for her sore muscles. Allowing herself the space to now deal with her mental health is giving her body time to heal. She now understands how mental health affects our physical bodies.

I had to face my fears, get out of my own way, and even admit I was afraid, not something I was ever okay with admitting. My larger-than-life self is always in your face to hide my fear of most things. Putting her away allowed me to see what I feared, deal with it, and push through it. I am worth that much.

This tribe has gone through the shittiest parts of life, as we all do. Things like divorce, loss, pain, joy, fear, illness, and fighting our way back from the dark. That is it, really. Finding a way to endure that crap, finding a way to get back up, and, more importantly, knowing we are worth finding joy in our new chapter of life.

You are worth it. You are worthy of laughing. You are worthy of being strong. You are worthy of happiness, regardless of age. So now, get out there and take what belongs to you.

What exactly do I want you to remember from this book? First, I want you to realize that strength training is a multifaceted discipline that requires dedication, discipline, and a scientific approach. Throughout this book, we have explored the fundamental principles of strength training, including the importance of motivation, proper form, and nutrition.

Additionally, we have discussed the importance of rest and recovery and the role of mindset and motivation in achieving success in strength training. While physical strength is undoubtedly an important part of strength training, mental strength and resilience are just as essential for long-term success.

Finally, it is essential to remember that strength training is not a one-size-fits-all solution. Everyone's goals, abilities, and limitations are unique, and it is vital to approach strength training with a personalized and individualized approach.

We cannot forget that it is a challenging and rewarding pursuit that improves our physical and mental health.

MUSCLES ARE SEXY

Reader, I want to take this time to speak directly to you. If you picked up this book because, like the tribe, you are a woman over 50 interested in strength training, hear this: There is no age limit on beauty. There is no age limit on strength. There is no age limit on ability, and there is sure as hell no age limit on sexy. You are driving your ship, and you can determine what works for you and feels comfortable. This advice I want to leave with you is that ability, not age, should determine every step of this next chapter in life for you.

I would like to ask that if you found any of the tips and advice in this book helpful, you leave a review on

Amazon. This allows me to spread the word on strength training to as many women as I can.

"I love this message, Franny. It reminds me of that first meeting we had with Marco and me admitting I was afraid strength training would make me bulky," Robbie remembers.

I do remember this conversation. He told us that strength training can actually help you build a strong, toned physique without necessarily making you look bulky. The idea that strength training automatically leads to unattractive muscle mass is a common misconception, but it's not necessarily true.

He continued to tell us that strength training can help you build lean muscle mass, which can actually improve your overall appearance by helping you look more toned and defined. Additionally, muscle is metabolically active tissue, meaning it burns more calories at rest than fat. Doing this will help you keep a healthy body weight and improve your health.

"Marco did such a great job of explaining everything, so I understood and leaned into my ability," Nora stated.

He wanted us to know that it's important to note that everyone's body is different and will respond differently to strength training. Some people may naturally build muscle mass more quickly than others. With the right approach and a focus on building lean muscle mass, strength training can help you achieve a strong, healthy physique that you're proud of.

"Man, I miss that guy. I never imagined in my entire life that I would say that about my trainer. He changed my entire perception of strength training," Robbie adds.

GOODBYE MARCO

The time has come. As much as the tribe and I have known this day would come, it doesn't make it any easier. Marco has become like family. He has celebrated our victories and held us up through pain and tears. We have thought long and hard about how to properly thank him. We know he is still building his clientele, and word-of-mouth advertising is everything in this business. So our tribe got together with Robbie via Zoom last night and gave Marco three of the best reviews possible to help boost his ratings. Outside of that, we did some great networking in our own circle to drum up some new business for him.

Nora and I show up for our final meeting with Marco. We greet him with a kind hug, tissues in hand. We tell Marco that there are not enough words and thank you's to express how we truly feel. Then, we quickly do a Zoom call to Robbie, knowing she doesn't want to miss our small surprise.

As soon as her face appears, she holds a sign with just the number 22. Marco asks, seeming a bit puzzled, "Hello Robbie, what are you all up to? I am a little confused."

I told Marco we didn't want to show up here with a cheesy thank-you gift, but we wanted to show our appreciation nonetheless. We had put our heads together last night and wrote three glowing reviews for him. Blushing, he thanks us profusely.

"But wait, there is more," I continue. "The number 22 is how many new clients we have found you."

"What?" He stammers, still wide-eyed.

"Marco, you have changed our lives forever and you are amazing at what you do," Nora chimes in. "We want to share your gift with as many people as we know," She continues.

"If you can handle the influx, they are ready." Robbie states, smiling with all her beautiful teeth.

Marco wraps his arms tightly around us, teary and laughing with gratitude. He blows kisses at Robbie, thanking her as well.

We wrap up our tearful goodbye and remind Marco; this isn't goodbye but a, see you soon.

NOTE FROM THE AUTHOR:

I hope you found my book to be an enjoyable and informative journey. As a self-help author, it is my passion to share not only my knowledge but also my personal story. I want my readers to know that they are not alone in their struggles and that the human factors of excuses and lack of motivation can affect us all.

When I set out to write this book, I wanted to do something different. I didn't want to simply provide information; I wanted to create a book that would inspire action. As I sat on my couch staring at my lifeless treadmill, I realized that so many of us buy exercise equipment with good intentions but end up using it as a clothes rack. So, I included some of the factors that could prevent the reader from taking action and provided strategies to overcome them.

My goal is to empower my readers to take control of their health and well-being. Together with my tribe sisters, we plan on writing three more books in this format with all of us on a health journey that we are dealing with together. I hope to inspire readers to join us on our journeys of self-improvement and personal growth.

I am deeply committed to helping women achieve their goals and overcome any obstacles that may stand in their way. If you found my book helpful, please consider leaving a review. Your feedback will help me to continue improving and creating content that resonates with my readers.

Scan the QR code to leave a review!

https://www.amazon.com/review/create-review/?
asin=B0CJL294KQ

For more information on the books we have published or plan to publish shortly, please check out our website: crazysisterspublishing.com. We are always happy to assist fellow women with books that help other women. If you have any ideas for a book you want to post, please go to the "contact us" page on the website:

CrazySistersPublishing.com

Perhaps you have a book you wrote and want to put on our website... contact us.

Thank you for taking the time to read my book. I hope it has inspired you to take action and make positive changes in your life. Remember, with a bit of motivation and determination, anything is possible.

Sincerely,

Francesca Russo

VIDEO RESOURCES

As I mentioned earlier in this book, I wanted to include a link to videos for excellent strength training videos for women over 50. However, I am aware many of us don't have access to gyms or trainers. For this reason, you will find a link to resources below to help.

Scan the QR code for training videos for women over 50!

https://crazysisterspublishing.com/exercise-videos/

RESOURCES

Allina Health's Public Health Department. (2000, October 1). *Before surgery hip exercises.* Allina Health. https://www.allinahealth.org/health-conditions-and-treatments/health-library/patient-educa tion/total-hip-replacement/preparing-for-surgery/before-surgery-exercise-program

American Diabetes Association. (n.d.). *Blood sugar and exercise.* American Diabetes Association. Retrieved February 25, 2023, from https://diabetes.org/healthy-living/fitness/getting-started-safely/blood-glucose-and-exercise#:~:text=Physical%20activity%20can%20lower%20your

Anderer, J. (2021, August 5). *Over 50? You should never exercise at this time of day, says science.* Eat This, Not That. https://www.eatthis.com/over-50-evening-exercise/#:~:text=Choosing%20to%20get%20your%20workouts

Atkinson, D. (2020, February 20). *How to get (and stay) motivated to workout after 50, 60 and 70.* Flipping Fifty. https://www.flippingfifty.com/motivated-to-workout-after-50/

Capritto, A. (2022, June 15). *How long does it really take to build muscle?* CNET. https://www.cnet.com/health/fitness/how-long-does-it-really-take-to-build-muscle/#:~:text=True%20beginners%20might%20see%20muscle

Carroll, J. E., Cole, S. W., Seeman, T. E., Breen, E. C., Witarama, T., Arevalo, J. M. G., Ma, J., & Irwin, M. R. (2016, January). Partial sleep deprivation activates the DNA damage response (DDR) and the senescence-associated secretory phenotype (SASP) in aged adult humans. *Brain, Behavior, and Immunity, 51,* 223–229. https://doi.org/10.1016/j.bbi.2015.08.024

CDC. (2020, July 27). *Osteoarthritis (OA).* Center for Disease Control and Prevention. https://www.cdc.gov/arthritis/basics/osteoarthri tis.htm#:~:text=Osteoarthritis%20(OA)%20is%20the%20most

Cleveland Clinic. (2020, July 29). *Don't make these 4 mistakes when you're lifting weights.* Cleveland Clinic. https://health.clevelandclinic.org/four-mistakes-avoid-lifting-weights/

Comprehensive Spine Institute. (2021, January 4). *Is weightlifting safe with osteoarthritis?* Comprehensive Spine Institute. https://www.c-siortho.com/blog/2021/january/is-weightlifting-safe-with-osteoarthritis-/#:~:text=Although%20it%20may%20seem%20like

Cramer, J., Weiss, S. (2018, December 18). *Why is it so hard for women over 50 to lose weight?* Northwest Community Healthcare. https://www.nch.org/news/why-is-it-so-hard-for-women-over-50-to-lose-weight/#:~:text=As%20we%20age%2C%20we%20lose

Cronkleton, E. (2019, July 18). *Try these 8 pool exercises for a full-body workout.* Healthline. https://www.healthline.com/health/fitness-exercise/pool-exercises

Mayo Clinic Staff. (2022, November 19). *Prediabetes - Symptoms and causes.* Mayo Clinic. https://www.mayoclinic.org/diseases-conditions/prediabetes/symptoms-causes/syc-20355278

Department of Health Services Victoria. (2012, January 6). *Empty nest syndrome.* Better Health Channel. Retrieved February 18, 2023, from https://www.betterhealth.vic.gov.au/health/healthyliving/empty-nest-syndrome

Eustice, C. (2023, February 7). *Weight training with osteoarthritis.* Verywell Health. https://www.verywellhealth.com/weight-training-with-osteoarthritis-4139960

Fit After Fifty. (2019, April 2). *Strengthen your willpower & motivation for fitness after 50.* Fit After Fifty. http://fitafterfifty.com/7-tips-to-stay-motivated-to-exercise/

Fitness 19 Team. (2021, July 23). *Is 72 hours enough for muscle recovery?* Fitness 19 .https://www.fit19.com/blog/is-72-hours-enough-for-muscle-recovery#:~:text=It

Forward. (2021, December 18). *How to lower your cholesterol with exercise.* Forward. https://goforward.com/blog/heart-health/how-to-lower-your-cholesterol-with-exercise#:~:text=Strength%20training%20

Freytag, C. (2022, November 17). *Weight training for women over 50: 11*

best moves. Get Healthy U. https://gethealthyu.com/strength-train
ing-moves-for-women-over-50/

Friedman, A. (2021, November 5). *Top 6 qualities of a successful strength and conditioning coach.* University of Denver. https://www.du.edu/
sport-sense/news/top-6-qualities-successful-strength-and-condi
tioning-coach#:~:text=The%20top%20six%20qualities%20that

Gordon, B. R., McDowell, C. P., Lyons, M., & Herring, M. P. (2020, October 16). Resistance exercise training for anxiety and worry symptoms among young adults: a randomized controlled trial. *Scientific Reports*, 10(1), 6–8. https://doi.org/10.1038/s41598-020-74608-6

HealthMatch Staff. (2022, May 11). *Taking vitamin D for seasonal affective disorder: All you need to know.* HealthMatch. https://healthmatch.
io/seasonal-affective-disorder/vitamin-d-for-seasonal-depres
sion#how-does-vitamin-d-help-with-seasonal-affective-disorder

Higuera, V. (2019, August 23). *The best exercises to lose weight and stay active.* Healthline Media. https://www.healthline.com/health/exer
cise-fitness/best-exercise-to-lose-weight

Kaiser Permanente. (2022, May 13). *7 surprising ways stress can affect your body.* Kaiser Foundation Health Plan. https://healthy.kaiserper
manente.org/health-wellness/healtharticle.7-ways-stress-affects-
body#:~:text=Stress%20can%20

Kamb, S. (2022, April 12). *5 travel workouts: Get in shape while traveling.* Nerd Fitness. https://www.nerdfitness.com/blog/how-to-stay-in-
shape-while-traveling/

Kassel, G. (2022, November 22). *Why you can't stop farting at the gym.* Health. https://www.health.com/fitness/workout-fart#:~:
text=Working%20out%20

Levine, H. (2022, December 12). *4 things we now know about hip replacement surgery.* Johnson & Johnson Services. https://www.jnj.com/
health-and-wellness/what-to-know-about-hip-replacement-
surgery

Liao, S. (2017, December 14). *Knee and hip exercises for osteoarthritis.* WebMD. https://www.webmd.com/osteoarthritis/features/oa-
knee-hip-exercises

Macha, A. (2017, April 5). *6 science-based secrets to staying motivated at the gym*. Better by Today. https://www.nbcnews.com/better/pop-culture/how-motivate-yourself-get-out-bed-work-out-today-ncna743006

MacPherson, R. (2023, January 25). *5 mental health benefits of strength training*. Verywell Fit. https://www.verywellfit.com/mental-health-benefits-of-strength-training-5216157#:~:text=Strength%20train ing%20can%20help%20our

Marturana Winderl, A., & Braithwaite, P. (2020, December 31). *Here's exactly how much water you should drink every day*. SELF. https://www.self.com/story/how-much-water-should-you-drink-a-day

Mayo Clinic Staff. (2021, August 21). *Osteoporosis - symptoms and causes*. Mayo Clinic. https://www.mayoclinic.org/diseases-conditions/osteoporosis/symptoms-causes/syc-20351968

Milkman, K. (2021, November 29). *How to build a habit in 5 steps, according to science*. CNN Health. https://www.cnn.com/2021/11/29/health/5-steps-habit-builder-wellness/index.html

NHS. (2017, October 23). *Osteoporosis - Causes*. Nhs.uk. https://www.nhs.uk/conditions/osteoporosis/causes/#:~:text=Women

Nunez, K. (2019, March 4). *11 diets from the 1980s that sound like hell on earth*. So Yummy! https://soyummy.com/1980s-diets/

Oerum, C. (2020, March 21). *How resistance training affects your blood sugar*. Diabetes Strong. https://diabetesstrong.com/how-resistance-training-affects-your-blood-sugar/

Roussy, S. (2022, July 5). *Best workout clothes for older women*. Sixty + Me. https://sixtyandme.com/best-workout-clothes-older-women/

Schroeder, E. C., Franke, W. D., Sharp, R. L., & Lee, D. (2019, January 7). Comparative effectiveness of aerobic, resistance, and combined training on cardiovascular disease risk factors: A randomized controlled trial. *National Library of Medicine*, 14(1). https://doi.org/10.1371/journal.pone.0210292

Stutz, J., Eiholzer, R., & Spengler, C. M. (2018, October 29). Effects of evening exercise on sleep in healthy participants: A systematic review and meta-analysis. *Sports Medicine*, 49(2), 269–287. https://doi.org/10.1007/s40279-018-1015-0

Tucker, A., & Sgobba, C. (2021, November 1). *How to find relief if your muscles are sore after a workout.* SELF. https://www.self.com/story/how-deal-post-workout-muscle-soreness-really-painful

Waehner, P. (2022, January 25). *Create a fitness mindset for workout motivation.* Verywell Fit. https://www.verywellfit.com/why-you-dont-exercise-1229953

Wheeler, M. J., Green, D. J., Ellis, K. A., Cerin, E., Heinonen, I., Naylor, L. H., Larsen, R., Wennberg, P., Borax Belk, C.-J., Lewis, J., Eikelis, N., Lautenschlager, N. T., Kingwell, B. A., Lambert, G., Owen, N., & Dunstan, D. W. (2019). Distinct effects of acute exercise and breaks in sitting on working memory and executive function in older adults: a three-arm, randomized cross-over trial to evaluate the effects of exercise with and without breaks in sitting on cognition. *British Journal of Sports Medicine,* 54(13). https://doi.org/10.1136/bjsports-2018-100168

Winternitz, W. (2016, March 11). *Hip replacement surgery rehabilitation exercises.* Arthritis-health. https://www.arthritis-health.com/surgery/hip-surgery/hip-replacement-surgery-rehabilitation-exercises

Made in the USA
Monee, IL
13 March 2024

54984969R00105